MIND NUTRITION

MIND
NUTRITION

TIMELESS SECRETS TO
ENHANCE YOUR BRAIN DAILY

BY JOSHUA EAGLE

CONTENTS

Introduction

The greatest gift we are given in life is that of our mind. When we properly nourish and guide our minds, we strengthen the force within us to cast our dreams into reality. In today's day in age however most have lost touch with this gift. Rather than seeking to uplift and strengthen their brain's most attempt to exploit and deplete them for short term gains and excitement through stimulants, pharmaceutical drugs and alcohol. If only they knew that much deeper states of joy and intelligence are found in working with the brain as an ally rather than an object to tap dry then perhaps we would treat the world in the same way. When our ancestors discovered the fact that no two brains are exactly alike, they were not only right in comparing two people to one another, but also in the respect that our own brains are not even identical to themselves from one second to the next. Modern technology has allowed us to look deeper into the mind, peering all the way down to the cellular level. What's been revealed is that our brains are continuously changing and can be guided to the heights of brilliance and creative genius, if only we so choose to lead them there. You may soon come to realize that there is no limit to how far the mind can evolve. No final boundary has yet been set. In this book I hope to give you the tools and knowledge to take your own mind on the path to ascended intelligence, deeper intuition and higher states of mental clarity than ever before experienced. I believe that everyone contains the potential for genius. Yet, in order to reach such heights you must first find the key to unlock it. Once the door is opened, the possibilities are infinite.

PART I:
FOODS FOR THOUGHT

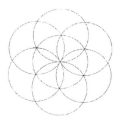

There may be nothing that has more of an influence over our minds than the foods we eat. Food acts as the foundation of the mind and raw materials used for constructing all of our brain cells, grey matter, neurotransmitters and neuronal wiring/connective tissue. Far more than just calories, the foods we are designed to eat have natural vibrant colors, flavors and life breathing nutrients which can transform our thoughts to a higher frequency. The old wives tale that we are only born with a set number of brain cells in life has been disproven time and time again. What's been shown rather is that the brain, like the body, is constantly regenerating itself, producing new brain cells and working to achieve it's pre-written destiny which lies encoded in our DNA. Captured in the double-stranded helices of our DNA are the blueprints for our own mind's complete and perfect physiological make up. This genetic design entails the instruction code for creating the perfect you and the perfect me. The keys to activating this perfection however lie in the attainment of the 5 Essences which have been recognized by all ancient civilizations since the dawn of humanity. In this section we will explore the 1st and perhaps most important essence impacting the mind, which is that of food.

A Drink For Zen Like Intelligence

One of the most powerful brain enhancing drinks ever discovered is that of Green Tea. While drinking Green Tea has been shown to benefit various different areas of overall health such as enhancing the immune system and fighting cancer, it is particularly valued throughout history for its power to supercharge and protect the brain. The most notable mind altering ingredient in Green Tea is the amino acid L-Theanine. Unlike certain energy drinks which put the mind into a state of jolted stimulation, the effects of L-Theanine work to put the mind into a state of calm mental alertness. The subtle effects of L-Theanine in Green Tea are so powerful that Buddhist monks seeking to enhance focus and relaxation during long hours of meditation traditionally use it as their drink of choice. As well as L-Theanine, Green Tea also contains a large amount of the substance EGCG. A study conducted at The University of Medical Technology in Taiwan showed that EGCG works to keep more neurotransmitters in the brain for longer periods of time by slowing the rate at which they are broken down. EGCG has also been shown to be a significantly more powerful antioxidant than vitamins C and E, and more than twice as powerful as the antioxidant Resveratrol found in red grapes. The antioxidant potency of Green Tea has been shown to protect brain cells as well as other areas of the brain such as the Hippocampus from toxins, free radicals and inflammation alike. Drink green tea in its organic loose-leaf form or by selecting high quality organic tea bags. For optimal health benefits drink 1-3 cups a day.

"Better to be deprived of food for three days, than tea for one."

-Chinese Proverb

"Tea tempers the spirit, and harmonizes the mind, dispels lassitude and relieves fatigue; awakens the thought and prevents drowsiness."

-Lu Yu (733-804)

"Who would then deny that when I am sipping tea in my tearoom I am swallowing the whole universe with it and that this very moment of my lifting the bowl to my lips is eternity itself transcending time and space?"

- D.T Suzuki

MUSHROOM OF IMMORTALITY

The most cherished mushroom in Chinese Medicine for a history of over 2000 years has been that of Reishi. Referred to in Chinese as the "Mushroom of Immortality," Reishi is valued for its powerful effects on sharpening the mind and improving focus, memory and consciousness. Found growing at the base of trees in mountainous areas near flowing springs, the Reishi mushroom is a rare find in nature. Due to its scarcity, in ancient times the mushroom was reserved for use only by the Chinese royal family and was considered to be more valuable than any jewel or precious metal. Chinese emperors became so obsessed with the Reishi mushroom that they would frequently send out thousands of people on quests to attain it for them. Certain Japanese folklore suggests that Japan was in fact founded by Chinese explorers on a mission to find Reishi for the Chinese emperor, yet rather than returning with the mushroom, chose to stay and colonize Japan. Since Reishi is considered to be a tonic, its benefits to the brain and body are cumulative in nature and can take one's mental and physical health to greater levels the longer it is consumed. In this understanding of Reishi, one could hypothetically begin taking the mushroom at age 30 and still be accumulating higher levels of benefit from the mushroom with every passing day they consume it. Although techniques for growing Reishi mushrooms have now been learned, it is believed that the most powerful Reishi's are those grown on wood similar to the trees they grow on naturally in the wild. Reishi can be drunk as a tea by simmering the mushroom in water for 1-3 hours. You may also choose to take Reishi as an alcohol tincture, or powder extract for it's adaptogenic uses.

Neuro-Transmission

Just as a computer relies on its Megahertz (MHz) for speed, our brains rely on neurotransmitters for thought processing, learning ability and feelings of happiness. The essential building blocks needed for our brains to build neurotransmitters are high quality proteins. However, while most people are taught that they need an overly excessive amount of protein to achieve optimal health, nothing could be farther from the truth. While protein is a fundamental component of life and nutrition, eating excess protein leads to large amounts of stagnant waste accumulation in the intestines, hardening of the arteries, kidney damage and makes one more susceptible to contracting infectious disease. While protein does play an important role in human health, one does not need to eat much of it to extract what is needed for a life of heightened vitality, health and joy. Vegetarians can seek out quality protein foods such as nuts, seeds, quinoa, blue-green algae, spirulina, bee pollen, goji berries and medicinal mushrooms for complete protein sources. For meat eaters, seek out organic sources of eggs, wild or grass fed meat, wild fish and organic free-range chicken. Aside from keeping our minds sharp and uplifted, neurotransmitters also work to ward off stress, depression and mental fatigue. Make sure you build them abundantly and remember that it's not the quantity of protein, but the quality that counts.

Serotonin	Vegetarian: Sunlight, Entheogens (see chapter 2), Goji Berries, Brazil Nuts, Almonds, Cashews, Avocado, Blue-Green Algae, Beets, Bee Pollen, Hempseed, Royal Jelly, Chia Seed, Honey, Hemp Seeds. Non-Vegetarian: Wild Fish, Grassfed Red Meat, Marine Phytoplankton, Krill Oil, Wild Game.
Dopamine	Vegetarian: Beets, Entheogens(see chapter 2), Mucuna, Apple, Wheat Germ, Organic Dairy Products. Non-Vegetarian: Eggs, Wild Fish, Chicken, Wild Game Meats.
Tryptophan	Vegetarian: Bananas, Spinach, Nuts, Broccoli, Asparagus, Bee Pollen, Chia Seeds, Brown Rice, Wild Rice, Entheogens(see chapter 2) Non-Vegetarian: Turkey, Eggs, Grass Fed Red Meat, Wild Fish.
Phenethylamine	Vegetarian: Cacao, Blue-Green Algae, Spirulina, Lentils, Nuts, Seeds. Entheogens(see chapter 2) Non-Vegetarian: Grass-fed Meat, Wild Fish.

GABA	Vegetarian: Green Tea, White Tea, Hummus, Kefir, Tomatoes. Non-Vegetarian: Wild caught Shrimp, Wild Fish.
Acetylcholine	Vegetarian: Grass Fed Butter, Avocado, Grass Fed Dairy Products. Non-Vegetarian: Eggs, Turkey, Wild Fish, Grass Fed Meat.
Glutamate	Vegetarian: Seeds, Organic Dairy Products, Non-Vegetarian: Grass-Fed Meat, Eggs, Wild Fish.
Glycine	Vegetarian: Seaweed, Blue-Green Algae, Spirulina, Watercress, Spinach, Sesame Seeds, Sunflower Seeds. Non-Vegetarian: Ostrich, Turkey, Eggs, Chicken, Grass Fed Red Meat.
Histamine	Vegetarian: Kimchi, Sauerkraut, Kefir, Kombucha, Spinach, Dates, Prunes, Figs.

A Red Rush To The Brain

One of the most powerful brain foods that has yet been discovered is that of Beets. The magic of this red root vegetable lies in its ability to boost blood flow and oxygen to the brain while simultaneously lowering one's blood pressure. The main antioxidant found in Beets is the amino acid Betaine. This compound works to increase levels of Serotonin and Dopamine in the brain which are key neurotransmitters responsible for maintaining a healthy mood and sense of well being. Betaine also works to enhance water retention in our cells and helps prevent dehydration so that our brains electrical functioning is more energetically conductive. Legendary philosopher and nutritionist Rudolf Steiner who was a huge proponent of Beets stated:

> *"The red beet stimulates thinking very strongly... but it does that in such a way that one actually wants to think. He who doesn't like to do this doesn't like red beets either."*

To get the most benefit, try juicing fresh organic Beets (uncooked). Since Beet juice is extremely detoxifying it is recommended that it is not drank alone, but rather mixed with other juices such as celery, cucumber, apple, carrot or others. Avoid canned beets since these varieties are often roasted and typically genetically modified as well as combined with hazardous chemicals and preservatives.

Liquid Crystal Intelligence

Ancient cultures throughout history have referred to water as being the source of all life. When taking a look into why so many towns throughout history included the word "spring" in them, we find it was because these civilizations were founded around springs which supported the life and health of the townspeople. In turn it is no surprise that high quality water is one of the key components in enhancing one's brain function. The human brain being comprised of 75% water is dependent on the substance not only for cell construction and blood flow, but also as a conductor of electricity. Water in fact is one of the most powerful conductors of electricity we have found to date in the universe and enables the brain to generate between 15-25 watts of power, enough to turn on a light bulb. Yet not all water is the same. The highest quality source of water one can drink is freshly gathered spring water from wild springs found embedded deep in nature. Unlike other forms of water, the molecules in wild spring water are arranged in billions of three-dimensional crystalline formations called tetrahedrons which enable spring water to receive, store and transmit vibrational and electromagnetic information. As well, the cleanliness and purity of spring water is far superior to well water, reverse-osmosis filtered water and carbon filtered water alike. Cut out the tap water, stop drinking bottled water and go straight to the source of life's magic, the spring.

*To find a spring near you visit www.findaspring.com

*For further information on living spring water please see Appendix A.

> "*The crystal has a very extensive memory. It remembers all the places it has been, all the people who have touched it and all the forces that have impregnated it. It is its molecular structure which gives it this particularity. Indeed, as you may know, minute pieces of crystal are used as 'chips' in computers and act as their memory.*"
>
> -Luc Bourgault

The Bible's #1 Brain Fruit

One of the best time tested foods for improving one's memory are Olive's. It may be no coincidence that the food is written about in the bible over 185 times! The main brain benefits from Olives come from their high content of Omega-3 and Omega-6 fatty acids which help insulate our brains and keeps them in top functioning condition. Yet this biblical fruit also contains many other healthful monounsaturated fats which work to keep the insulation of our brain cells as well as nerves intact and at proper production levels. Since the brain is around 60% fat, maintaining healthy fats in one's diet is an essential component for keeping the brain at proper functioning. Consumption of Olive's has also been linked to greater production of cell energy (ATP) and may help to protect the body from diseases such as Cancer, Alzheimer's and other conditions. One can choose to eat olives in a variety of different ways from eating regular whole organic Olives to using Extra Virgin Organic Olive Oil. Just 1-2 tablespoons of organic olive oil a day or 3-7 olives can bring you great benefits. Seek out Olives which are organic and have not been pitted and exposed to oxygen.

LIVING VITAMINS

Living vitamins are those which are derived from foods which were once alive. Whether ingested from fruits, vegetables, animals, herbs or the sun, these vitamins contain their full spectrum of supporting nutrients and compounds that make them biologically absorbable by the body. Vitamin pills however, which are nearly all currently synthetically created in laboratories, are not only less absorbable by the body, but can harm our health and lead to a host of illnesses and disorders. Along with frequently containing numerous pesticide sprayed and genetically modified ingredients such as maltodextrin, absorbic acid and others, the minerals found in these synthetic vitamins are frequently found to be produced from ground up inorganic rocks as well as other Earthly substances not meant for ingestion. Since superior brain health is dependent on having quality bio-absorbable vitamins, seek them out in their whole food form, or in whole food organic supplements and bypass all chemical imitation vitamins in the process.

LIVING VITAMINS INDEX

Vitamin A	Carrots, Yams, Spinach, Kale, Cayenne, Mustard Greens, Collards, Swiss Chard
Vitamin B	Bee Pollen, Eggs, Meat, Honey, Kombucha, Wheat Germ, Comfrey, Clams, Oysters, Mussles
Vitamin C	Green Tea, Oranges, Rose Hips, Camu Camu Berry, Bell Peppers, Strawberries
Calcium	Spinach, Collard Greens, Seeds, Orange Pithes, Nuts, Avocado
Vitamin D	Sunlight, Wild Salmon, Medicinal Mushrooms, Sardines, Eggs
Vitamin E	Avocado, Sunflower Seeds, Pine Nuts, Almonds, Swiss Chard
Vitamin K	Green Tea, Kale, Spinach, Dandelion Greens, Swiss Chard, Broccoli
Magnesium	Sage, Basil, Dill, Chives, Spearmint, Corriander, Wheat Germ, Pumpkin Seeds, Cacao or Dark Chocolate, Sesame Seeds, Sunflower Seeds, Nuts, Rye, Oats, Buckwheat

NATURE'S SWEETEST MEDICINE

Honey is food that is produced by Bee's that convert the nectar of the flowers they visit into this sweet sticky yellow treat. Honey's history of use in medicine dates back to ancient times in both religion and throughout countless cultures. On top of being a highly nutritious food containing an abundance of antioxidants, amino acids and polyphenols, Honey also contains numerous properties which work to benefit brain health. One of honey's foundational ingredients is Glucose which acts as the primary source of fuel for our brain's energy. Glucose in Honey works to ensure that activities such as thinking, learning and memory retention are working at full capacity. As well, Glucose ensures that our brain has the energy needed for neurotransmitter production and synapse communication. Also found in Honey are critical brain supporting vitamins such as B1, B2, B3, B5 and B6 which all play unique roles in brain development and repair. When choosing a honey seek out locally, wild harvested or organic varieties. Never consume non-organic honey since pesticides can become concentrated in the wax produced by these bee colonies and is shown to leach into all areas of the bee's hive. For B vitamins, go to the Bee's.

THE #1 ANIMAL BRAIN FOOD

Animal foods are not a necessity for reaching ascended states of mind nutrition and can sometimes actually be detrimental to this, however if one does happen to be a meat eater, as most people are, than no animal food may be more healing to the brain than that of wild fish. Considering that our brains themselves are comprised of almost entirely water and fat, it is no coincidence that this fatty water animal is a perfect brain match. The main ingredient in wild fish that makes it such a powerful brain food is its high level of *long chain* Omega-3 fatty acids. Unlike seeds and nuts which contain only short chain Omega-3 fatty acids, wild fish contains high amounts of long chain Omega 3's which provides both key brain hormones EPA and DHA to the brain. EPA and DHA are both essential building blocks for producing brain cells, neurotransmitters, and our myelin sheaths that coat and protect our nerves. Proper amounts of EPA and DHA may be even more important for pregnant mothers and the elderly who require higher amounts of these ingredients to aid growing and aging brains. For high quality wild fish packed with Omega 3's look towards sockeye salmon, black cod, sardines, mackerel and herring, always wild.

MUSCLE UP YOUR MEMORY

Ginkgo Biloba has an extensive history of use as a brain-boosting herb which dates back thousands of years to ancient China. While the Ginkgo leaf has long been held as a memory enhancement supplement in Traditional Chinese Medicine, it is just recently being valued amongst western cultures as a valuable brain enhancing food as well. The Ginkgo leaf extract has been shown to enhance blood flow as well as oxygen utilization in the brain and proves to be a potent antioxidant and free radical scavenger as well. Brain benefits of Ginkgo can include improved long and short-term memory, increased mental clarity and improved reaction time. Take Ginkgo in its organic powdered form by adding 1-2 teaspoons of it to smoothies, teas or soups. You can also choose to seek out Ginkgo in its organic extract form. *Avoid Gingko supplements sourced from China as recent testing has shown these supplements to contain high levels of neurotoxic heavy metals.

POISON IN THE WELL

One of the most dangerous chemicals our society is faced with today is that of Fluoride. Unlike the organic form of Fluoride found in nature, synthetic fluoride is a potent neurotoxin and is currently being added to the majority of public water supplies, toothpastes and antidepressants. Fluoride's first use in water came about by the Nazi's in World War II concentration camps where they found it to produce a mind numbing effect on the prisoners, suppressing their will power and making them subservient and docile. The Nazi's may have gotten this idea due to the fact that Fluoride has been used as a main ingredient in rat poison since the 1800's. The dangers of fluoride are gaining more attention as new studies are turning up that specifically reveal fluoride's damaging effects to the brain. A recent study out of India concluded that exposure to fluoride is directly correlated to reduced intelligence in children and revealed that as the level of fluoride increased in the child, the level of intelligence decreased. Yet equally as bad as fluoride's damaging effects on intelligence is the recent discovery that it is also found to concentrate around and encrust the brain's pineal gland. This is problematic considering the pineal gland is responsible for producing the key neurotransmitters serotonin and melatonin and is responsible for regulating sleep/wake cycles. The Pineal Gland is also assigned sacred value in Buddhism, Hinduism, and Taoism, which all refer to it as being, "the third eye" chakra and believe that if trained correctly it can perceive senses beyond physical sight. To protect yourself from fluoride, avoid ingesting tap water, toothpastes and other products that have fluoride added to them. Your third eye will thank you.

Enhance Your 2nd Brain

Most people don't understand the role our gut plays in maintaining a healthy mind, but scientists often refer to the stomach as our, "second brain". The reason for this is due to the fact that it actually contains roughly 100 million neurons, as well as 500 million nerve cells. Not only does our stomach communicate with our brain chemically and electrically, but it also produces neurotransmitters such as serotonin which works to help regulate our mood and state of emotional well-being. In fact, the greatest quantities of Serotonin in the body are not found in the brain, but are actually found in the intestines. By maintaining a healthy level of probiotic bacteria in our stomachs we not only work to enhance our bodies serotonin production, but also help to protect our stomachs neuronal network and ensure it can communicate effectively with our brain. In a 2011 study it was shown that by enhancing probiotic bacteria levels in mice they experienced decreased anxiety, enhanced central nervous system functioning and improved communication between the brain and stomach. To enhance your levels of probiotic flora start by adding organic fermented foods into your diet such as Kimchi, Sauerkraut, Kombucha and or Kefir. You can also chose to take an organic food based probiotic supplement which can also help enhance your bodies levels of probiotic flora.

Ancient Aztec Food of the Gods

Chocolate is not only one of the best desserts in the world, but the cacao bean, where all chocolate comes from, is also one of the best foods you can consume for your brain. The key to Cacao's magic lies in its mineralization. In order for the brain to run effectively it must have the proper amount of essential minerals present. A lack of adequate minerals in the brain can easily lead to neurological disorders, ADD, ADHD and general cognitive problems. This is where the Cacao Bean comes in. Contained in the Cacao bean are the highest found food sources of Magnesium, Iron and Chromium. Likewise, Cacao also contains extremely high quantities of Manganese, Zinc and Copper. The amounts of minerals found in Cacao are so abundant in fact that one could choose to use it as a replacement for their mineral supplement entirely. Last but not least, Cacao also contains powerful neurotransmitters such Phenylethylamine and Anandamide which work to enhance feelings of bliss and give your mood a boost. To get to most benefit from Cacao, eat the beans raw or in their organic powdered form. Cooked chocolate will not provide as much benefit since heat can destroy Cacao's vitamins and antioxidants. When choosing a Cacao product seek out the 100% Arriba Nacional variety as this is the original strain of Cacao derived from the wild.

When In Doubt, Leave Out

What did Jesus, Moses, Buddha, Socrates and and the ancient Egyptians all have in common? Answer: They all engaged in the practice of fasting. In turn it may be no surprise that one of the best time tested ways to improve mental clarity and rejuvenate the brain is through partaking in a fast. Our digestive systems are constantly being bombarded by the food we eat throughout the day, and as a result are often playing a never ending game of catch-up to eliminate old food and digest new food. In this state of constant digestion our bodies are never given a chance to rest and detoxify properly. When a fast is finally undertaken, a massive weight is taken off of the body which frees up large amounts of energy. This new energy is used to produce Human Growth Hormone (HGH) which stimulates the production of new brain cells and neurons. A study out of Intermountain Medical Center showed that people who partook in a 24 hour fast had between a 1300% to 2000% increase in Human Growth Hormone as a result. The biggest brain benefit from fasting however may be provided as a result of the detoxification that occurs during a fast. Since the body no longer has to work to eliminate new toxins, it is permitted to backtrack and clean up older stored toxins that have compiled in the brain and body throughout the course of a persons lifetime. Accumulated waste such as synthetic chemicals, heavy metals, pesticides and other toxins can then be further eliminated from the body as a result. One who is new to fasting can begin by skipping a meal during the day. From there a person can move onto juice fasting and eventually spring water fasting. People suffering from disease or on medication should always consult a physician before partaking in a fast.

THE WORLD'S MOST COMPLETE FRUIT

The Avocado is a fatty fruit that has been dubbed by some as being the world's most perfect food. Avocado's work to promote brain health by providing an abundance of key nutrients including vitamins A, C, D, E, K as well as numerous B vitamins. The most notable brain nutrients found in Avocado's however are their omega 3 rich mono-unsaturated fats. These healing fats work to enhance good cholesterol (HDL) production while decreasing bad cholesterol (LDL) levels. The end result of this is lowered blood pressure, which in turn enhances cognitive functioning by boosting blood flow to the brain. Studies have also shown the fat found in Avocado's to protect the nerves in our brains from free radical damage. This protection is noted to be of particular benefit to the brain's prefrontal cortex which is responsible for tasks such as critical thinking and planning. To benefit from Avocado's eat anywhere from a quarter to a whole one per day.

SLEEP SMARTER

If you're looking for an herb that can help you get to sleep at night while improving your brain health simultaneously, then look no farther than Skullcap. Originally given its name due to its flowers resemblance of a skull protecting helmet, Skullcap appears to do just that, protect your head! A unique ingredient found in Skullcap known as Baicalein has been shown to help protect the brain against a type of oxidation related to brain diseases such as Parkinson's and Alzheimer's disease. As well, a second unique ingredient in Skullcap known as Oroxylin has been shown to improve symptoms of ADHD such as hyperactivity, impulsivity and poor attention span. Skullcap is a great alternative to pharmaceutical sleeping pills. To make a nighttime Skullcap tea, steep a tablespoon of organic Skullcap in hot water for 3-5 minutes and drink at your own pace. Avoid taking Skullcap if you are pregnant.

The Healthiest Food Of All

Foods that are harvested from the wild are always found to be higher in antioxidants, vitamins and minerals than food grown by man through farming and gardening. The reason why these foods contain higher amounts of nutrition is because the same ingredients which are healthy to us are what these plant's use as defense weapons to guard themselves against diseases, predators and pests. Since these wild plants need to fend for themselves without help from man, they evolve to develop stronger nutritional properties which in turn makes them healthier foods to eat. Yet along with being extra nutritious, wild foods are also shown to have a powerful effect to strengthen our DNA on a cellular level. What's been revealed is that the genetic information contained in the DNA and RNA of all plant foods works its way into our own human DNA when eaten. Since the genes contained in wild foods are the strongest of all, by eating more of them we can introduce this superior genetic information into our own bodies DNA. Wild foods such as berries, greens, mushrooms and for non vegetarians wild game meats, can all make valuable additions to one's diet. While wild foods are indeed the highest form of nutrition on our planet, one should always make sure to correctly identify all wild foods before eating them, as some can be poisonous.

WILD FOOD RECOMMENDATIONS

Wild Greens:	Dandelion (flowers, greens and roots), Lambs Quarters, Prickly Lettuce, Seaweeds, Nettles, Chickweed, Purslane, Mallow, Pine needles(tea)
Wild Berries	Blueberry, Raspberry, Blackberry, Strawberry, Bilberry, Cherries, Mullberries, Serviceberries, Gooseberries, Hackberries
Wild Fruits	Coconut, Sea Grapes, Prickly Pear, Crab Apples,
Wild Mushrooms	Reishi, Chaga, Shiitake, Maitake, Ganoderma, Birch Polyore, Fomes Fomentarius, Morel, Chantrelle
Other	Wild Rice, Fiddleheads, Maple Syrup, Wild Honey, Wild Asparagus, Birch Syrup, Sea Salt, Spring Water

* Always make sure that you identify any wild food you find and know 100% positively that it is edible and not

poisonous, particularly with ground mushrooms. For wild food foraging book recommendations see Recommended Reading.

Turns out, the Garden of Eden wasn't really a garden at all.
It was anything but a garden: jungle, forest, wild seashore, open savanna, wind blown tundra. Adam and Eve weren't kicked out of a garden. They were kicked into one.

-Christopher Ryan

"I am tired of this thing called science… We have spent millions on this sort of thing for the last few years and it is time it should be stopped."

-Senator Simon Cameron, 1901

"It is especially difficult for modern people to conceive that our modern, scientific age might not be an improvement over the pre-scientific period."

- Michael Crichton

Tiny Brain In A Shell

It may be no coincidence that the appearance of the Walnut resembles the same design shape as the human brain. A plethora of studies are now compiling which show the direct benefit to brainpower from consuming these omega-3 rich nuts. One recent study on Walnuts showed a significant improvement in learning abilities and memory retention in male rats that were fed walnuts for a period of 28 days. The rats were also observed to navigate maze challenges more efficiently than their non-walnut fed competitors. Further analysis into the brains of these walnut fed rats revealed that the rats had developed increased serotonin neurotransmitter levels as well as 5-HTP levels. This author recommends selecting whole walnuts which have not been removed from their shells and exposed to open air. This is to ensure the walnuts have maximum freshness as well as retention of their brain benefiting nutritional properties.

GMO's

Just as the DNA from healthy foods can work to strengthen our own genetic intelligence so too can the altered DNA of genetically modified foods (GMO's) work to harm our health and DNA. GMO foods come from seeds that have been tampered with by scientists so that they cannot reproduce and on the contrary, will commit suicide. Corporations have altered the DNA of GMO foods in this way so they will not create new seeds and the farmer will have to buy them again the following year. Adding further problems to GMO's is the fact that they are created to be heavily sprayed with poisons such as pesticides and herbicides which the GMO companies also sell. This makes it so the consumer is not only eating food which has been genetically altered to commit suicide, but has also been soaked in toxic poison throughout it's life and grown in demineralized soils. In a study published in the International Journal of Biological Sciences it was revealed that mice fed a diet of GMO foods developed numerous tumors, severe organ damage and 70% of the females died prematurely. To avoid GMO's eat as organic as possible and be mindful of the top GMO foods currently grown such as corn, soy, sugar, beets and canola.

FERMENTED FOODS

Eating foods such as Kimchi, Sauerkraut, Kefir and Kombucha, which are rich in probiotic bacteria can not only boost your mood, but may also make you more intelligent as well. What's been found is that the good bacteria living on these foods actually produce large amounts of neurotransmitters in our bodies which are then released into our bloodstreams. Feel good neurotransmitters such as GABA, Serotonin, Dopamine, Norepinephrine and Acetylcholine have all been shown to be produced by these probiotic bacteria and can help improve overall mental health as well as nervous system functioning. Add fermented foods into your meals and snacks regularly and let your bacteria allies go to work.

LIQUID VITALITY

Aside from providing a massive detoxification to the body, juicing organic vegetables and fruits further provides enormous energy and invigoration to the mind and body. Being that everything which we eat eventually gets liquefied by the body in order for our foods nutrients to be absorbed into the walls of our intestines, juicing works to free the body from having to do extra work as it provides pure liquid nutrition directly into our living cells. In the juicing process, toxins as well as negative energy stored in our tissues becomes flushed out rapidly and in proportion to the length one remains on a juice diet. This at first can cause a person to experience fatigue, irritability and even depression as these toxins are purged out of the body. After initial sensations of discomfort our pushed through however, the true magic of juice fasting becomes apparent as ones body becomes enlivened by the natural photonic light energy which the juiced plants have absorbed through photosynthesis. In working with juicing one should look to consume low sugar juices which are primarily green plant and chlorophyll rich based. More acidic juices are recommended earlier in the day as these can work as a natural soap to the gastrointestinal tract from which the drawn out toxins can then be pushed out later in the day through the neutralizing and washing effect of green juices. Since juicing requires a level of dedication and self-discipline it is recommended that one begin on their juice journey in steps and stages. One can start by merely replacing one meal of their day with juice instead of solid food. From there one can gradually build up to juice fasting one day and then multiple days. Begin a juice cleanse today and free yourself from toxins and stagnant energy that can weigh you down physically, emotionally, mentally and spiritually.

THE HUMAN PLANT

Of all the Chinese herbs to ever exist, there may be none more ferociously hunted for in the America's than that of Ginseng. The name Ginseng translates in Chinese to the word "man" and was given this name due to the roots similar resemblance and appearance of a human being. The power of the Ginseng root comes from the plants ability to live in the ground for hundreds of years where it lays gathering energies from the Earth, forest and stars. From this energy the plant goes on to produce what are known as Ginsenosides. These Ginsenosides have been shown in studies to have a major effect on brain functioning and enhance areas of attention span, learning ability, thought processing and memory retention. The Ginseng Extract has also been shown in animal studies to stimulate brain cell activity and help regenerate damaged brain stems in animals. Perhaps it is no coincidence that Ginseng has been used for thousands of years in Chinese medicine to help counter the effects of aging on the brain and to restore youth and vitality to adults. To benefit from Ginseng, make a tea by simmering 25-35 grams of Panax Ginseng Root in a pot of water for 5-15 minutes. You can also choose to take Ginseng in its organic capsule extract, or powdered form through adding it to smoothies or tea.

Fire Up Your Circulation

Aside from being a delicious spicy food, Cayenne peppers can also be used to help fire up your brain cells. Found in this hot pepper is a unique antioxidant called Capsaicin which when digested works to open up our blood capillaries and allow more nutrients to be drawn into our bloodstream. Animal studies reveal Cayenne's ability to help protect the brain by shielding brain fats from breakdown as well as protect brain cells from injury and damage from certain chemicals. To get the benefits of Cayenne's firepower, add it as a chopped up raw or as a powdered spice to soups, entrees and salads alike.

The Best Tasting Vitamin Yet

Goji Berries, also known as Wolfberries, contain a store-house of vitamins, antioxidants and polysaccharides which work to both enhance and protect the brain. Packed into these tiny berries are over 30 trace minerals such as calcium, iron, zinc, and 19 amino acids which are essential for optimal brain health. The use of Goji Berries dates back over 2000 years when they were first recognized as being a "Superior Tonic" in China's first Herbal Encyclopedia. As well as preserving youth and overall health, recent studies show that Goji Berries also work to protect our brain cells, enhance learning capacity, and improve memory retention. A recent study from the University of Hong Kong concluded that Goji Berry Extract provided neuro-protective effects against certain neurodegenerative diseases, in particularly Alzheimer's. The Goji Berry Extract not only protected brain neurons from harmful toxins, but was also shown to contain powerful anti-aging properties as well. To best benefit from Goji Berries, seek them out in their dried, fresh, or juiced form.

B Vitamins = Brain Vitamins

The family of B-Vitamins are an essential component for maintaining a healthy brain and nervous system. Not only are B-Vitamins shown to help alleviate symptoms of depression and ward off brain shrinkage, but they also work to support brain development and proper energy production. Three foods which act as powerhouses for a variety of B Vitamins are those of: Wheat Germ, Kombucha and coincidentally, Bee products.

1. Wheat Germ which has often been referred to as, "the staff of life" is actually found to contain the entire B vitamin complex along with numerous enzymes, vitamins and minerals as well. While bread produced prior to 1840 included the wheat germ in it, current bread has the wheat germ removed to extend its store shelf life. Unfortunately this process removes the very magic that bread was eaten for since the days of biblical times. The bible which makes numerous references to "unleavened bread", refers to wheat germ in Deuteronomy stating, "the LORD alone did lead him...and he made him to suck honey... with the fat of kidneys of wheat." To get the benefits of wheat germ use it in it's organic supplement form, or seek out a bread maker who still makes it the original and intended way, stone ground with the wheat germ intact.

2. Kombucha which is a fermented probiotic drink hailing from China contains a host of brain strengthening B-Vitamins including B1, B2, B3, B6, B9 and B12.

The probiotic bacteria contained in Kombucha also works to help build neurotransmitters in the body, detoxify the liver and decrease levels of harmful bacteria throughout the body and brain. Since harmful bacteria have been linked to anxiety, pain, cognition and depression, flooding the body with good probiotic bacteria helps to rebalance your body's bacteria levels and support overall brain and central nervous system functioning.

3. Bee Products such as Bee Pollen, Honey and Royal Jelly are not only rich sources of B-vitamins, but are also found to contain all the essential components needed for life.

Bee Pollen, which is made out of millions of microscopic flower particles gathered by bee's, allows us to take in all of the beautifying ingredients which flowers are made of. These flower essences are not just the embodiment of beauty however, but are found to contain 40% of the highest quality bioavailable protein in nature. Adding to this are also Bee Pollen's ingredients of vitamins A, C, D, and K, more amino acids than beef and extremely rare trace minerals. So rare are some of the unique minerals found in Bee Pollen that to this day scientists are not able to identify or synthetically replicate them.

Royal Jelly is the food reserved exclusively for queen bees of the colony. The potent vitamins, rare fatty acids and antibacterial proteins in this super-honey are just some of the ingredients which allow the queen bee's to develop their much larger brains and bodies. Recent studies on the properties of Royal Jelly have shown its power to stimulate new brain cell growth, improve memory, learning and even turn on genes in our RNA to protect the brain. Seek out Royal Jelly products in their organic and least processed form and mix with honey or a smoothie for best taste.

Insulate Your Brain With This Healthy Fat

Coconut oil is the gelatinous substance that can be extracted from the meat of the Coconut fruit. The oil is shown to contain certain fatty acids including lauric acid which gives the food powerful antiviral, anti-bacterial, anti-microbial and anti-fungal properties. Coconut oil is found to breakdown into what are known as Ketone bodies which in turn are believed to supply an alternative source of energy to brain cells which can no longer run on glucose. New research is further suggesting that Coconut Oil may also be an effective supplement in working to prevent neurodegenerative diseases such as Alzheimer's. Seek out coconut oil products in their organic and least processed form and add them to smoothies, hot drinks or desserts for best tast.

HEAVY METAL: GOOD MUSIC, BAD FOOD

Heavy Metal toxicity is a problem that is becoming ever more prevalent in our industrialized world. While metals can do a decent job in making certain products and machines, they are extremely harmful to human health and can wreak havoc on the brain. The most common heavy metals that can damage brain functioning are mercury, aluminum, lead, arsenic and cadmium. The result of ingesting these metals can range from a list of various ailments including: reduced IQ, brain damage, dementia, disorientation, impaired motor functioning and neuron damage. A study conducted at Arizona State University revealed that children with Autism on average had much higher levels of toxic metals showing up in their blood and urine samples. To help avoid ingesting heavy metals seek out food that has not been grown with pesticides, aluminum free deodorants, organic cosmetics and aluminum free cookware. Meat eaters should avoid eating fish that are larger in size since these fish have a tendency to accumulate higher levels of mercury being that they are higher on the food chain. Last but not least, if you've ever received mercury fillings in your mouth please consider having them professionally removed. Foods that can help detoxify heavy metals from your body are garlic, onions, cilantro, radish, spring water, zeolite clay and bentonite clay.

SOUTH AMERICAN WONDER DRINK

The South American tea known as Yerba Maté is loaded with high quantities of antioxidants, minerals and amino acids which work to stimulate energy in the brain. Commonly used in South America to fight fatigue, Yerba Maté tea is known to provide energy similar to that of Coffee, but with less of the jittery side effects. The unique ingredients found in Yerba Maté that provide its energy boosting effects are called Xanthines. These unique compounds not only work to stimulate the brain's functioning, but also simultaneously provide a calming effect, reducing feelings of stress and anxiety. Yet that's not all, a recent animal study using a Yerba Maté extract revealed the extract to improve short-term memory as well as social memory in its recipients. To prepare Yerba Maté, make a tea using 1-2 tablespoons in an organic unbleached bag or loose-leaf form, steep for 5 minutes and enjoy.

CHOLINE: A STRONG FOUNDATION HOLDS THE KEY

A key nutrient that plays an essential role in building a strong memory and mind is Choline. A study conducted at the Duke University Medical Center showed that pregnant female rats that were fed Choline while pregnant gave birth to offspring with apparent "superbrains". These newly born rats not only displayed increased neuron connectivity, but also showed superior memory retention and ability to learn new tasks which lasted with them throughout their lives. What makes Choline such a valuable brain nutrient is it's needed supply in order to produce Acetylcholine which is a neurotransmitter responsible for memory. Choline is also required as a foundational material used by the brain in order to produce nerves and neurotransmitter receptor sites. The best food sources of Choline include nuts, broccoli, eggs and fish. You can also choose to organically supplement with choline by taking an organic supplement with 450mcg for women and 550mcg for men.

Herbs of Elasticity

When it comes to building and reinforcing the crystalline structure of your bones, joints, ligaments and nervous system, the duo of Stinging Nettle and Horsetail tea is perhaps the most powerful formula around. This anti-inflammatory brew works to provide your body with an abundance of the essential mineral silicon (silica), which is the precursor necessary for your body to manufacture bioavailable forms of calcium. Furthermore, the phytochemicals found in this tea act as both a diuretic and astringent, working to help purify the blood as well as aid in respiratory, digestive, and neuronal-connective functioning throughout the body. Yet on a level pertaining to physical aesthetic health and beauty, the combo of Horsetail and Nettle tea throws in a much appreciated gift in through acting as a precursor to collagen production, hence increasing the bio-elasticity of our connective tissue, skin, hair and nails. To make Horsetail and Nettle Tea simply steep 1-2 tablespoons of each herb in a cup or pot of hot water for 10-30 minutes, let cool and drink.

Star Berries

Of all the colors found in food, the rarest encountered is that of blue. The Native Americans knew this fact, which could be why they highly valued and readily consumed the fruit of Blueberries. Admiring the berries for their star shaped tops, Native American's referred to Blueberries as "Star Berries" and used them for both food and medicine. Since that pastime, science has confirmed the medicinal benefits of Blueberries and revealed the fruits ability to sharpen memory, boost brain cell communication and flush the brain of toxic chemicals. The secret ingredient in Blueberries which gives them their blue color is an antioxidant known as Anthocyanin. Numerous studies on Anthocyanin show its effects to shield the brain from aging as well as reduce oxidative stress from smoking and alcohol. While all types of Blueberries are shown to benefit the brain, wild blueberries are shown to have the strongest brain benefits packing twice the amount of antioxidants as conventional Blueberries. To add Blueberries into your life, try incorporating them into your breakfast, salads and especially desserts. They not only help your brain, but taste great too.

BRAIN DETOX DELICACY

The use of Garlic dates back 7,000 years to ancient China and Egypt where it was traditionally used as both a food and medicine. As well as containing numerous antibacterial, antiviral, antifungal and antimicrobial properties, recent studies show that consuming Garlic also enhances our brain functioning. In a study conducted at the Tufts University School of Medicine, mice that were fed an aged garlic extract showed increased cognitive functioning, improved memory and enhanced longevity. A further study conducted at the Medical University of South Carolina showed that compounds in Garlic worked to effectively destroy brain cancer cells and tumor cells alike. A potent anti-inflammatory food, Garlic works to detoxify both the brain and body. Those looking to benefit from the numerous healthful properties of Garlic may choose to consume it in meals, as an organic extract or in its powdered form.

FAKE FLAVORS

Artificial flavorings such as MSG, and artificial sweeteners are shown to be neurotoxic and physically destructive to the brain. Studies show that these ingredients not only kill brain cells as well as nerve cells, but can also lead to addictive cravings to consume more of these artificial flavor ingredients. Likewise, consuming these ingredients has also been shown to lead to obesity in animal studies. To avoid dangerous artificial flavorings make sure you read the ingredients list in the foods you purchase. Foods that can frequently contain MSG as an ingredient are pre-made soups, fast food meals, potato chips and various snacks, processed foods and condiments. Foods likely to contain artificial sweeteners are diet sodas, chewing gum, mints, candies, frozen yogurts and coffee flavorings. Commonly these dangerous ingredients will go by different names or brand names such as Splenda™, Equal™ or Nutrasweet™. Make sure you're knowledgeable of what you're eating and if you can't pronounce it, you should probably do without it.

NEUROTRANSMITTER ROCKET FUEL

One of the most powerful neurotransmitter producing foods yet discovered is that of Mucuna. This vine like plant has a long history in Herbalism and natural health for being used to help conditions ranging from neurological disorders sucha as Parkinson's disease and for easing stress. Mucuna itself is shown to contain neurotransmitter chemicals such as Serotonin, L-Dopa and 5-HTP which work to boost mood and improve ones sense of well-being. These neurotransmitters are also key components for brain cell communication which can make the computer of your mind run faster and more efficiently. Mucuna is most commonly consumed in crushed or powdered form where it is then added to drinks or desserts. Anywhere from a teaspoon to a tablespoon added to a drink can have a profound effect in uplifting your mind and mood.

THE OMEGA-3 SEED

Chia seeds have been long hailed in Central and South America as a dense source of nutrition and energy producing food. The Aztecs, Mayans and current day Tarahumara Indians all consumed Chia Seeds for the healthful benefits they provide. The area of our body which sits to best benefit from this tiny food however is none other than the brain. Although small, Chia Seeds contain a high quantity of Omega-3 Fatty Acids which work to enhance and protect our minds. Chia Seeds contain an even higher quality of omega-3 oil's than fish, and don't carry the risk of containing numerous toxins and heavy metals which are turning up more frequently in our fish and meat supply as a result of pollution. Along with a high quantity of omega 3's, Chia Seeds also contains 19 amino acids, numerous antioxidants and are a complete protein source. Chia Seeds can be eaten in a variety of different ways. Add the seeds to smoothies, salads, oatmeal, or just about any dish you like. You may also consume them in the traditional Tarahumara Indian drink called, "Iskiate" by simply adding a tablespoon of Chia Seeds to your cup of water and letting the seeds sit for 15 minutes to a few hours before drinking. Since Chia Seeds have the ability to gain more than 10 times their weight by absorbing water, Iskiate was consumed to help prolong hydration as well as electrolyte retention for the active lifestyle endured by the indigenous Tarahumara people.

The Answer In The Ocean

If you travel all the way to the very bottom of the food chain, you will arrive at a food which may be the foundation of all mental cognition across the planet. This food is no other than Marine Phytoplankton. NASA estimates that this particular ocean plant is responsible for producing between 50% to 90% of the Earth's oxygen. That is more than is produced by all of the forests and trees on the Earth combined. As a brain food Marine Phytoplankton packs a powerful punch per weight. It is a complete protein which contains all 10 essential amino acids needed for proper brain function and also contains a potent quantity of omega-3 fatty acids. In fact, just 1 oz of Marine Phytoplankton contains roughly 400mg of the Omega 3 fatty acids, an essential component for proper brain functioning. Yet there are even more nutrients found in Marine Phytoplankton. Further contained in this powerful food are several B Vitamins as well as minerals such as magnesium, calcium, zinc, copper, manganese, iodine, potassium and sodium, which work to support optimal brain health.

PICK YOUR BRAIN UP WITH THIS
SOUTH AMERICAN BREW

Drinking Coffee has been shown to provide many benefits to our brain as well as overall health. A drink rich in antioxidants, studies have shown Coffee to help fight off free radical damage as well as protect against Alzheimer's and Depression. A study of 1,400 longtime Coffee drinkers in Finland showed that people in their 40's and 50's who drank 3-5 cups of Coffee per day were 65% less likely to develop Alzheimer's Disease than those who consumed less than 2 cups per day. As well, another Coffee study conducted on rats showed that rats that consumed Coffee in their diet had improved long-term memory, concentration and object recognition. Since coffee does have a high caffeine content which can become addictive, it is recommended that one drink coffee in moderation no more than 2-3 times a week. When choosing a Coffee brand this author recommends picking one which has been certified organic and works with fair trade standards.

• People prone to nervousness, anxiety, or who are suffering from neurological conditions such as Parkinson's or Alzheimer's disease should avoid Coffee as it can overly exhaust dopamine levels in the brain.

SHIELD YOUR BRAIN WITH THIS INDIAN HERB

One of the most prized herbs from the Indian system of Ayurvedic medicine is the stress fighting plant known as Ashwagandha. The power of Ashwagandha comes from its naturally contained steroids and alkaloids which work to protect our brain cells from free radical damage and counteract the harmful effects of stress on the nervous system. Ashwagandha has also been shown to enhance memory and help rebuild neuronal networks in the brains animals suffering from certain neurodegenerative diseases such as Alzheimer's and Parkinson's Disease. To get the benefits of Ashwagandha consume 3-6 grams in a tea or organic powdered extract form. Powdered extracts can be added to smoothies and tea's for best taste. A little bit goes a long way.

STIMULATE YOUR PINEAL GLAND

On top of being extremely high in antioxidants and a potent natural antibiotic, the Indian root Tumeric is also one of the best brain boosters and detoxifiers found in the grocery store. Prized in the Middle East and Asia for over 5,000 years, Tumeric has been shown to help fight a host of mental disorders such as Alzheimer's, depression and anxiety. During a study conducted at The University of Singapore led by Dr. Tze-Pin Ng, test takers who consumed Tumeric prior to test taking showed significantly higher scores on the Mini Mental State Examination when compared to the study participants who did not consume Tumeric prior to testing. Yet on top of Tumeric's brain boosting powers, the specific anti-inflammatory compound found in Tumeric known as Curcumin has been shown to detoxify the brain by helping to cleanse it of accumulated heavy metals and toxins such as aluminum, mercury, fluoride and iron.

For further in depth guidance on activating your pineal gland please see Appendix C.

IF MAN MADE IT, DON'T INGEST IT

Since the 1940's humans have introduced over 75,000 new toxic chemicals into the planet. These chemicals are known to cause a host of health problems such as brain damage, nervous system disorders, cancer, organ damage and other issues. Avoiding these chemicals entirely has now become impossible due to the fact that they have worked their way throughout our entire planet's ecosystem. Not only are babies umbilical cords now found to contain over 200 industrial chemicals and pollutants, but even polar bear cubs as far as the north pole are now found to have PCB chemicals from plastic showing up in their fatty tissue. Do your best to avoid exposure to toxic chemicals by choosing natural and organic products over synthetic and toxic ones and remember, if man made it, don't eat it.

THE DYNAMIC DUO

The two chlorophyll rich herbs Cilantro and Parsley are a great pair to help clean out heavy metals and toxins from the brain and bloodstream. Cilantro, which is rich in vitamin A and K works to naturally thin the blood and reduce bad cholesterol levels. From there parsley comes in with vitamin C, beta-carotene and high amounts of chlorophyll to help drive toxins through the liver and out of the body. Pair these two plant allies in salads, soups, juices, smoothies and side dishes to help to banish brain toxins away today.

BLUE GREEN MAGIC

One of the most nutrient dense foods on the planet, blue-green algae in its organic or Spirulina form provides a host of vitamins, minerals, complete proteins and long chain Omega-3 fatty acids to keep your brain in tip-top shape. Perhaps the best source of complete protein for those on a vegan diet, what makes blue-green algae such a special food is the fact that up to 97% of its vitamins, enzymes, and 65 trace minerals are easily absorbed by our bodies due to their high bioavailability. Responsible for providing blue-green algae its bluish color is its high quantity of AFA cyan probiotic bacteria, which bestows stem-cell producing and repairing abilities as well as acts as a source of the hard to come by vitamin B12. However, further contained in AFA is the compound Phenylethylamine which is a natural brain chemical that when produced induces states of mental clarity, well-being and bliss. Blue-green algae is a great addition to smoothies, green tea and medicinal mushroom tea. Mix them all together to unlock even greater magic.

HERBALISM

Herbs are one of the true sources of medicine handed down to us from nature. In working with them, they can act to teach our body and mind through educating us with their own unique plant phytochemical ingredients. By consuming a wide variety of herbs, we can learn from a wide variety of teachers. Though the classroom exists on a cellular level, and lessons are taught in a language without words, the results can be experienced through subtle physiological changes over time. As all herbs contain their own unique properties, some are found to have a special affinity for that of the mind. Incorporate medicinal herbs into your daily life one at a time, seek out new ones that call to you, and see where your path unfolds.

> *"What is a weed? A plant whose virtues have not yet been discovered."*
> –Ralph Waldo Emerson

> *"One of our greatest fears is to eat the wildness of the world. Our mothers intuitively understood something essential: The Green is poisonous to civilization. If we eat the wild, it begins to work inside us, altering us, changing us."*
> -Stephen Harrod Buhner

Part II
THE MIND IN MOTION

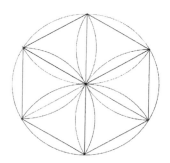

The human body is just a smaller, holographic reflection of our Mother Earth. Just as the Earth's oceans, rivers, and springs flow life into the veins of our planet, so too do our own bodies propel blood and lymph to hydrate and nourish our own inner ecosystem. As the Earth breaths air and vitality into all of its plants, animals and landscapes, so too do our own lungs and veins deliver oxygen and life force to our own inner universe of cells, tissues and organs. In this cycle of nourishing and cleansing, the quality of our body's fluids, matter and air are as essential to our being and radiance as the purity of the oceans, forests and atmosphere are to the Earth's. When the energies brought by water and air in their natural harmonic state are combined with the essences of Food and Sunlight in theirs, what is born is what ancient cultures referred to as The 5th Essence. Recognized by the Chinese as "Chi", the Greeks as, "Aether", the Hindus as "Prana" and the Polynesian's as "Mana", this invisible state of energy which can exist in us all, can only be brought to life through the proper unification of the 4 Elements; Air (Oxygen), Earth (Food), Fire (Sunlight) and Water in their pure natural living states. In this section we will look at ancient, time tested techniques for bringing to life the 5th Essence and reaching the next level of universal intelligence and harmony.

ILLUMINATE YOUR MIND

The sun is the supreme giver of all life and the greatest source of energy existing in our solar system. The receiving of sunlight not only works to stimulate the mind, but is also held as one of the 5 essential elements in Traditional Chinese and Indian medical philosophies. Just as water is the source of all life, the Sun is the source of all water. For it is not until the hydrogen radiating from the sun merges with the oxygen of the Earth's atmosphere that water (H_2O) can be born. The sun which delivers a male energy to our mother Earth, is also responsible for stimulating our bodies to produce the essential brain antioxidant Vitamin D. Our bodies naturally produce Vitamin D when the sun's UVB light reacts with the cholesterol in our skin and Vitamin D is absorbed directly into our bloodstream. Studies on Vitamin D show its powers to enhance our brain by supporting information processing speed, reducing memory loss and potentially helping to prevent various neurodegenerative diseases. Yet the sun provides much more to our brains than just Vitamin D. By exposing different parts of our bodies to sunlight, we trigger different biological responses in the body. For example, exposing the male reproductive area to the sun is shown to multiply hormone levels in men by up to 300%. Likewise, exposing areas of our face and head to sunlight stimulates our brains pineal and hypothalamus glands to produce neurotransmitters which support overall mental functioning. The idea that people have been led to see the sun as a destroyer of health rather than a provider of it will be looked back on as one of the greatest health myths ever pulled on our generation. Don't run from the sun, embrace it, and allow the spark to ignite in the flame of your mind.

Grow Your Brain

If you're looking to literally grow your brain larger and stronger, then perhaps you should start meditating. Scientific research from Harvard and MIT on long-term meditators shows their brains to grow significantly larger in areas responsible for learning, memory, concentration and emotion. Meditators brains have also been shown to have increased brain-cell connectivity and thickness when compared to those of non-meditators. The research shows that the longer a person has been meditating, the larger their brain size becomes. As well, meditation is also revealed to significantly increase one's levels of intelligence, creativity and sense of intuitive perception. In a university study on 100 college men and women it was shown that those who meditated for a period of two years improved significantly on intelligence tests when compared to those who did not meditate. Since part of the benefit of meditation comes from oxygenating the brain, it is beneficial to meditate in areas with clean, fresh air. The best way to learn how to meditate properly is by attending an in person meditation class and receiving personal instruction. You can also choose amongst the countless great books, audio recordings and videos available on the subject. More important than how you learn, is that you do learn. Commit today, and embark on your path to a higher state of consciousness.

Tap Into This Invisible Energy

Air is the breath of life, the messenger of spiritual awakening and the pathway of consciousness. Just as plants need the purest air in order to grow to their strongest potential, so too does your brain. The founders of Chinese medicine understood this fact, which is why they listed Air as being one of the essential five elements needed for superior health. Yet the Chinese weren't referring to just any old air floating around. They were specifically speaking of living air that is filled with oxygen. You can find this air in forests, mountains, coastlines and wherever trees and greenery are abundant. If your environment is devoid of these oxygen-producing plants then your air is likely to be low in oxygen and lacking vitality and energy. As well as the Chinese, the ancient Yoga masters of India also realized the power of oxygen, which is the reason why they created a practice called, "The Yogic Breath". To complete the Yogic Breath start by finding a place where you can breathe fresh oxygenated air. Begin by inhaling through your nose for a period of 8 seconds. Hold this breath for 16 seconds and then exhale out through the mouth for a period lasting 12 seconds. Repeat this process seven times for best results. In practicing the Yogic Breath you will be strengthening your lungs in the same way that a weight lifter strengthens their muscles. As your lung capacity increases, so too will your ability to draw in and absorb the mind enhancing energies of living oxygen.

Your Second Life

Your level of alertness and clarity throughout the day is directly impacted by the quality of sleep you receive at night. Getting enough sleep is not only your birthright, but is also a vital necessity to ensure that your brain can run at full capacity. People who receive adequate sleep at night are shown to have improved memory, attention span and learning capacity. On the other side, poor sleep is linked to mental issues such as ADHD, depression, bipolar disorder, schizophrenia, low immunity and anxiety. The National Sleep Foundation recommends adults receive between 7-9 hours of sleep at night, but everyone is different. Determining your own sleep needs through assessing your personal feelings upon waking is important to take note of. To maximize the healing and re-charging of your brain during sleep there are a number of techniques that exist. The best is to first open a window in your room at night and allow fresh air in. Since we evolved from ancestors who originally lived and slept outdoors, recreating a similar environment by letting outside air in not only helps to oxygenate our minds while we sleep, but can allow us to experience a past time in history when people lived and slept in fresh air 24 hours a day. A second step to take is to make sure the room you sleep in is dark and quiet. Since our brain releases the sleep hormone melatonin as a result of darkness, avoiding lights and electronic device screens at night can help get your circadian rhythm attuned to the Earth's natural day/night cycle, where the only lights in existence are those of the stars and moon.

Step Outside The Box

Spending time in nature can deliver an experience of peacefulness and freedom to those who seek it. By stepping out into wild forests, mountains, beaches and other natural landscapes, we can re-experience the magic of our planets natural environment and tap back into the real world we once came from. The absence of linearity in nature such as those of straight roads, perfect angled buildings, and grid shaped cities, re-awakens an area of our brain that is rarely used in these modern times. This area is that of the original mind. In stimulating this original mind through establishing a relationship with nature, we begin reconnecting to our deeper levels of sensory perception of that around us. This area of perception is often blunted and overloaded by the constant activity carried on around us in urban settings. When unlocked however, our minds can experience new doors of heightened awareness allowing for deeper consciousness to emerge, and the intelligence of our wild planet and universe to enter.

Secrets of The Soil

While most people try to avoid getting dirty, numerous scientific studies now show that ingesting soil as a result of inhalation or by accident can drastically improve brain functioning. What's been discovered is that a specific strain of bacteria in soil called, "Mycobacterium Vaccae" stimulates brain cells to produce large amounts of the neurotransmitter serotonin, and can provide an antidepressant like effect. This type of soil bacteria is of course not harmful and is referred to as "friendly bacteria". Studies conducted on mice who were fed peanut butter mixed with soil, as well as a study on mice injected with soil bacteria revealed the mice to complete maze tests twice as fast, display less stress and anxiety, and have better concentration and learning ability than average. To add more of these friendly soil bacteria into your life, take up gardening, go out hiking or simply get outside more. If you have kids, take them to play in grassy fields or out in nature rather than cemented playgrounds and indoor game rooms. Dirt is not just good for the brain, but is also the main ingredient which allows oxygen producing trees and food bearing plants to live. Get back out into the dirt and uncover the most abundant brain secret here all along, right under your feet.

ELECTRIFY YOUR MIND

Throughout most of our history on this planet, rather than insulating our feet from the Earth by wearing shoes, humans walked barefoot with a constant electrical connection to the ground. Not only are our bodies shown to discharge energy to the ground when in direct contact, but more importantly they are also shown to draw in electricity and antioxidants which are constantly being released from the Earth's surface in the form of electrons. Unfortunately in wearing shoes we cut ourselves off from this powerful source of health which not only confuses our minds circadian rhythm, but also promotes inflammation and oxidation in the brain and body. Having our skin in direct contact with the Earth on the other hand has been shown to enhance electrical conductivity in the brain as well as reduce levels of the stress hormone Cortisol. To get more of the beneficial healing effects from the Earth and increase the flow of electricity to your mind, get your skin into direct contact with the Earth as much as possible. Activities such as going to the beach, taking off your shoes in the park, or doing yard work barefoot are just a few ways you can act to re-expose yourself to the healing energies of the Earth you are naturally designed to receive.

INCREASE YOUR EQ

Aside from just making your physical body more flexible, the practice of Yoga can also significantly increase a persons level of EQ. Similar to a person's IQ which measures one's mental intelligence, a persons EQ refers to one's emotional intelligence. This emotional intelligence entails a person's strength in their ability to form relationships, control personal emotions, tap into deeper states of intuition and perceive the emotions of others. A study out of India revealed that participants who practiced Yoga for only 5 days managed to increase their EQ levels by an average of 72%. The idea that Yoga not only makes one more flexible physically, but also increases one's mental and emotional flexibility is a core principle in yogic philosophy. Yet the brain benefits of yoga don't end with just EQ. Since yoga incorporates many postures where the head is below the heart, these inverted positions cause gravity to drive blood and oxygen to the brain, freeing up stagnation that may be present in the neck and head. To begin practicing Yoga, start by taking a class in person or on video. The original and most studied form of Yoga is called Hatha Yoga or "Sun/Moon Yoga". Begin with this traditional style and branch out to newer variations after if interested.

COSMIC INTELLIGENCE

In the early years of humanity the original form of night-time entertainment wasn't a TV show or movie, but rather was the act of stargazing. While this activity may sound uninteresting or boring to some, there is a deeper experience involved in viewing stars other than just spotting constellations. In peering out into the depths of the naked universe, every star we see transmits a unique harmonic light frequency. When these light frequencies enter into our eyes, the light continues to travel through our optic nerves until reaching an organ in our brain called the pineal gland. The pineal gland has been referred to throughout time as being our, "third eye". This is because when dissected our pineal gland is revealed to contain photoreceptors identical to those of our two actual eyes. As our pineal gland receives these distant light transmissions, it is stimulated to conduct it's job of producing neurotransmitters which in turn work to enhance our speed of cognition and overall sense of well being. Early civilizations would assign the practice of stargazing to religious priests so they could fulfill their mission in understanding the divine heavens. To gain your own cosmic intelligence step outside on a starry night and let your star journey begin.

Ditch The Pillow

Have you ever wondered why people use pillows? As it turns out, the first recorded use of pillows was in ancient China where they were made to assist birthing mothers, aid elderly men and be sold to the wealthy. Yet when placing pillows under our heads, they may do more harm than good. Aside from bringing on possible problems such as neck pain and breathing obstruction, pillows can also work to impede blood flow and oxygen to the brain while we sleep. Since we spend nearly 1/3 of our lives sleeping, the negative impacts from pillow use can add up over time. Rather than sleeping on pillows which kink our necks upward, try sleeping in a natural position that feels most comfortable to you. Such positions can include sleeping on your side, chest, or stomach with your head turned to one side, or just sleeping plain flat on your back. Like any habit, pillows can certainly be addicting, so ditch your pillow slow and allow your brain to return to flow.

TAKE THE PLUNGE

The most bone chilling practice ever carried out by our ancient ancestors of Europe, Asia and India was an act known as the cold plunge. The idea was simple. Find the coldest body of water you can come across, strip down, and jump in. Such was the thought in Siberia where those seeking natural highs and enhanced health took it upon themselves to jump full on into lakes and pools formed by melting glaciers. Since that time the scientific research has come to verify the health benefits of cold water therapy, and revealed it's particularly powerful effects on the brain. What's been shown is that as our skins nerve receptors make contact with cold water, electrical impulses are sent out to our brain which triggers a release of endorphins and neurotransmitters. By exposing our whole bodies to cold water we can stimulate an antidepressant like effect which boosts our mood and is also shown to improve learning performance. The best way to embark on a cold plunge is to start of with warmth. Try sitting in a sauna, going on a hike or doing some exercise to heat up. From there you can either take a cold shower, jump in a lake, or if you're very adventurous, find a melting glacier.

Smarter in 30 Minutes

If you're looking for an exercise that can make your smarter in just 30 minutes, then look no farther than running. Along with providing an exhilarating rush of feel good endorphins, running has also been shown to actually grow your brain. The act of running stimulates growth in an area of the brain known as the Hippocampus which is responsible for learning, memory and organization. Running has not only been shown to increase the size of the Hippocampus itself, but also resulted in significantly improved memory recollection as well. Perhaps this is also related to the fact that running is shown to stimulate the growth of up to hundreds of thousands of new brain cells, and increases the production of grey matter in the brain. Yet if that wasn't enough, there's still more. The act of running also works to boosts blood flow and oxygen to the brain, leading to increased cognitive speed as mental awareness. For those looking to maximize the benefits of running try running in outdoor fresh air settings such as parks, nature preserves or sandy beaches. Running on soft surfaces such as grass or sand will also serve to provide a softer running surface to help protect the knees and spine.

Digging Deeper

Negative emotions such as stress and past traumas are frequently absorbed into different parts of the body where they can manifest as knots, tightness, inflexibility or pain. In alleviating the body and mind of these physical ailments the best avenue to take is seeing a skilled deep tissue massage practitioner who may specialize in areas such as Rolfing, Swedish Massage, deep tissue massage or Shiatsu. These forms of deep tissue massages allow for practitioners to work aggressively into areas of your body which can often be holding accumulated stress and negative emotions. The act of deep tissue bodywork cracks open these negativity storage vaults of the body and allows for relief as well as energy and blood flow restoration by physically driving them out. To expand even further into deep tissue massaging benefits one can visit a hot spring retreat center where the combination of bodywork and hot spring therapy will multiply the positive healing effects.

MUSIC OF THE MULTIVERSE

If you asked a Quantum Physics professor about the nature of our universe, they would likely tell you about String Theory, of which the underlying foundation is actually music. If you asked a plant the same question, it would likely tell you nothing, because plants don't talk. However, if to that plant you played the music of Bach, Beethoven or other classical musicians, you might find that the plant grew faster, stronger and blossomed in the direction of the music's source. Such was the case for plant researchers Dorothy Retallack, Arthur Locker, George Smith and countless others whom all discovered this reaction from plants that were subjected to classical music. Likewise, a similar find was made by Japanese researcher Dr. Masaru Emoto who discovered that when water is exposed to classical music its molecules re-organize into star like shapes and symmetrical patterns viewable under a microscope. So what does this all have to do with the brain? In terms of our mind, what's been revealed across the board is that listening to music you enjoy improves brain functioning on multiple levels. Not only is listening to music you love shown to stimulate the brains entire neural circuitry, but it has also been shown to help strengthen the connection between the right and left hemispheres of the brain responsible for our creative and mathematical trains of thought. Further shown has been music's ability to stimulate creativity by shifting the brain into Alpha and Beta wave states which promote relaxation, mental clarity and imagination. Listen to the music you love while exercising, driving, or just being, and tune your brain to the endless harmonies of the universe.

"Cosmos: (Greek Origin) A single harmonious system."

THE BEST BRAIN DETOX

One of the most effective and time-tested ways to cleanse the blood, brain and body of harmful toxins is through the use of a sauna. Similar to showering which works to cleanse the body on an external level, using a sauna works to cleanse the body from the inside out. What makes sweating in a sauna such an effective detoxification tool is that not only are water soluble toxins such as pharmaceuticals, chlorine and synthetic chemicals excreted from the body, but fat-soluble toxins such as radiation, heavy metals and PCB's from plastics are also eliminated from the body via our pores. These fat-soluble toxins are more difficult to eliminate due to the fact that they accumulate in our fatty tissues where they typically remain stagnant. Through the act of sweating however we can draw these toxins out and up to the surface of our skin where we can wash them away afterwards. While many forms of exercise are also a good way to sweat, detoxification only happens minimally during exercise. This is because as a result of the physical stress placed on the body during exercise, the sympathetic nervous system is activated which works to prepare our body for defense against a perceived threat. This activation of our sympathetic nervous system directs our energy towards increasing our heart rate, producing adrenaline and other biodefense mechanisms. Sweating in a relaxed state such as in a sauna however does not activate this fight or flight response, which allows our body's energy to be directed towards healing and rejuvenation. Last but not least, sweating through the use of a sauna provides a massive relief to our body's liver and kidneys as it takes the detoxification burden off of these organs and allows toxins to be drawn out directly from our blood.

The benefits of sauna can be gained whether you use an electric sauna, wood fired sauna, infrared sauna and especially a traditional Native American sweat lodge. The key is to be relaxed and sweating. Try using a sauna 1-4 times a week for 20-30 minutes at a time for best results. If you are on medication please consult with your doctor prior to using a sauna as drugs are typically drawn out of the body to varying degrees when using a sauna. Do not use a sauna if you are pregnant.

Kundalini Energy

Activating your greatest energetic potential referred to as the Kundalini, is an invaluable gift which everyone should attain in life. The Kundalini is a universal life force energy which flows upwards from the base of the spine, rising through our 33 vertebrae and chakra points, until eventually reaching the top two energy points in our head known as the pineal gland and crown chakra. To activate the Kundalini to its highest point in the spine involves breaking through all energetic blockages within the bodies chakra system so that the energy can be conducted up the spine to it's highest point in the head. The spine, like all bones of our body is in fact technically a crystalline structure. This is because the molecular arrangement of our bones are of a tetrahedral geometric organized matrix and act as conductors of piezoelectric electromagnetic energy. The activation of one's Kundalini while rarely occurring spontaneously, typically involves the consistent engagement in a disciplined energy practice the likes of Kundalini Yoga, Ba Gua, Tai Chi or Chi Gong. One could even practice several of these modalities and enhance their Kundalini's evolution even further. Once attained, the Kundalini is a wellspring of high vibrational energy which assists one in all aspects of their life physically, mentally, emotionally and spiritually. Begin working to cultivate your Kundalini energy today and experience the greatest heights of your energetic self.

Internal Martial Arts

While our mainstream culture has become drawn into the various physical forms of martial arts used in televised fighting, a much less physically destructive and esoteric form of cultivating the internal force of fire within can be found in the ancient forms of Chinese internal martial arts. These art forms consisting of Ba Gua, Tai Chi, Neigong, Chi Gong and others, stem from the ancient Chinese Taoist quest for immortality. The foundational component to each of these modalities is to use the human body and mind as an electrical extension chord to cultivating internal energy from our external surroundings including the ground, air and ethers, so that we may harness this energy in abundance and use it at will. In situations where self-defense is required, the internal arts practitioner can transfer this internal energy into their opponent similar to plugging an electrical device into a power socket. Working with universal energy in this manner as well as in the yogic practices enables one to generate greater mental focus, physical energy and will power to direct one's efforts in the ways in which they choose. The breath work and flowing motions of these art forms further instills states of peace and tranquility which carries on with one in their daily lives. Those interested in working with forms of internal martial arts should attend beginner classes of various forms and see which type resonates most with them on a personal and energetic level.

Expressing The Shadow Self

In working to generate greater internal fire within while simultaneously purging out expressions of our own darkness which may be clogged within us, a very clear cut and direct method which should be utilized is that of external martial arts. Engaging in art forms of physical combat forces us to physically step out of our shells and express our pent up darker emotions which many fail to release in our everyday lives. This shadow self within us all, if not addressed can manifest in the form of physical illness, low energy levels, complacency and being easily manipulated and swayed due to lack of personal will power. In working to physically express this shadow self which can contain emotions such as resentment, anger, regret, shame, shyness and the like, the act of physically aggressive exercise such as external combat pushes the body to energetically expel these darker aspects of ourselves through physical exudence. Forms of external martial arts recommended for both working with our shadow self and cultivating fire are kickboxing, jiu-jitsu and the vast library of other offensive combative art forms in existence.

LEVITY

While the theory of gravity is widely known and accepted, very few give notice or have been taught about the force of Levity. The idea of levity was first brought forth by German philosopher Johan Goethe who stated that while gravity explained how an apple fell from a tree's branches, it failed to answer the more challenging question of how it got up so high in the first place. The power of levity can be seen in all aspects of nature, from water evaporating and rising up as clouds, to trees blossoming and falling upwards towards the sun. In terms of our brains, levity plays a much greater role than gravity by assisting the heart to deliver nutrients and oxygen upwards via our blood. While gravity works to slow blood flow to the brain through pushing it downwards, we have learned ways to flip gravity, turning it from a toxin into a medicine. The best ways of reversing gravity are through doing inverted Yoga postures, or by using an inversion table. Yoga which incorporates many positions of inversion, allows the head to be placed below the heart, reversing the forces of gravity and levity and sending greater blood flow to the brain. Likewise, a piece of modern day exercise equipment called an inversion table allows for one to flip themselves upside down with ease, releasing compression of the spine and assisting blood flow to the brain. Understanding the counterbalance between gravity and levity is an important concept to keep in mind as we tend to live in a world which fails to see things full circle. Use the forces of levity and gravity to your advantage a few times a week and help send further levitative properties to your brain.

PART III
POWER PLANTS

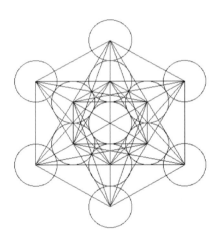

ENTHEOGEN:

(Oxford Dictionary)
From Greek, literally 'becoming divine within'.

ENTHEOGEN:

(Latin Translation)

En - *To cause a person or thing to be in.*

Theo - *A combining form meaning "God," used in the formation of compound words.*

Gen - *That which generates or produces.*

INTRODUCTION

Throughout the study of natural health and nutrition it becomes quite evident that specific plants work to heal and address specific parts of the body. We see that plants such as Dandelion Root, Burdock Root and Yellow Dock Root are evidenced to help heal aspects of the liver. Likewise, plants such as hawthorn berry, cacao beans and the oil of olives, coconuts and avocados all help to help heal aspects of the heart and cardiovascular system. The various medicinal mushrooms of the world such as Chaga, Reishi, Maitake and Shiitake in turn are shown to heal and correct imbalances and deficiencies of the immune system and its corresponding cellular matrix. While this book has already gone over specific foods that address brain health and mind ascension, there is no category of food which exists that is more powerful for healing and strengthening the mind than that of the power plant family, otherwise known as Entheogens.

Where Entheogens specifically come into play is in their ability to penetrate the blood brain barrier and introduce potent medicinal alkaloid compounds as well as rare phytochemicals which stimulate the regeneration, synchronization and detoxification of our brains synaptic chains, neurons, energetic wiring, brain cells and corresponding hemispheres. Simultaneously these plants further work to stimulate the brains pineal gland which is responsible for producing neurotransmitters and hormones such as Serotonin and Melatonin.

In specific cases where people are suffering from dis-biotic (unfriendly) bacteria and or parasites which have infiltrated the brain, it is very difficult for the body to hone in on attacking and removing these pathogenic organisms because of the protective structure of our bodies blood brain barrier. Bacteria can enter the brain through numerous avenues, but are far more capable of entering the brain when a trauma to the head has taken place in which the skin of the head has been broken or the head has been hit so hard that the blood brain barrier has been compromised. When the skin of the head is exposed open air through a wound, bacteria can then directly enter the brain through bypassing the blood brain barrier. This is why cancers such as Glioblastoma (brain cancer) are of the most deadly forms of Cancer types and typically require surgical procedures on the head in order to introduce so called medicines to the brain. The following pages discuss what I believe to be the most powerful mind healing and brain ascension tools that have yet been discovered to this day and how they work to heal and strengthen the mind.

Ayahuasca

∞

Ayahuasca is a South American tea that is made from boiling the bark of the Ayahuasca vine and the leaves of the Chacruna plant. Contained in the leaves of Chucruna is a highly medicinal and psychoactive natural compound called Dimethyltryptamine (DMT) which when combined with the Ayahuasca bark is allowed to be absorbed into the body and bloodstream. Countless studies on Ayahuasca have shown its potent abilities to heal people from various different illnesses and diseases, but in particularly Ayahuasca has revealed its extreme power to heal people from mental and emotional issues such as depression, anxiety, fear, and overcoming past traumatic events.

On a biological level Ayahuasca works to strengthen the brain by creating new synaptic chains, neurotransmitter receptor sites and synchronizing imbalances in the brains various hemispheres and neuronal wiring. Ayahuasca also works to detoxify the brain as the tea contains potent methyl donors and unique alkaloids that work to clean out toxins and debris which have accumulated in the brain such as synthetic chemicals, heavy metals, fluoride and other impurities.

In scientific studies conducted by Dr. Jordi Riba and his staff researching Ayahuasca's effects on the mind, Ayahuasca was shown via medical imaging to hyper-activate the brains neo-cortex, which is responsible for higher human functioning tasks such as perception, reasoning and decision-making. Ayahuasca was also shown to activate the brains Amygdala and Insula which are areas responsible for storing early childhood memories, past traumatic events and creating a bridge between our emotional memories and decision making. Typically when a new stimulus enters the brain, the brain tries to understand it based on our past experiences. Early traumatic events in life typically create an imprint or pattern in the brain which acts as a shortcut that becomes activated every time we face a similar situation. For example, if during one's childhood they were attacked by a dog, their brain might retain a pathway that associates that dog to all dogs and cause them to react with extreme fear whenever they see or hear any dog. Ayahuasca allows the conscious part of the brain to override these past traumatic events and heal a person from these burdensome fears.

Being that Ayahuasca works on a physical, mental, emotional and spiritual level, it is common for people who partake in Ayahuasca ceremonies to report their life's purpose being revealed to them while under the influence of the tea. It is also common for people to report gaining insights into the true issues in their way from achieving their goals and mission in life. Those interested in partaking in Ayahuasca tea ceremonies should seek out a reputable Ayahuasca Center with excellent reviews. One should never drink Ayahuasca tea without an experienced and trustworthy Shaman to administer the tea and guide the Ayahuasca ceremony.

San Pedro

San Pedro is considered a sacred cactus in South America where it has been used in traditional Andean medicine and religious divination ceremonies for over 3000 years. San Pedro in English translates to the name Saint Peter who was one of Jesus's 12 apostles said to hold the keys to the gates of heaven. In turn, ancient South American cultures also believed that through the responsible consumption of San Pedro under the guidance of a trained shaman, one could reach Heaven while still here on Earth. In the indigenous South American Quechua language the word for San Pedro is "Punku" which in English translates to "doorway".

The San Pedro cactus contains over 30 rare medicinal alkaloids such as organic mescaline and several other organic neurotransmitters which when properly consumed pass through the blood brain barrier and work to heal and strengthen the mind, body and spirit. As San Pedro goes into effect it specifically works to detoxify, heal and regenerate areas of the brain responsible for sensory perception such as sight, hearing, smelling, feeling and last but not least, intuition. San Pedro also specifically works on the cardiovascular system via detoxifying and strengthening the hearts circulatory networks and arteries. In regards to bacteria and parasites, San Pedro is shown to rigorously destroy pathogens living in the brain, heart and blood due to its powerful antimicrobial ingredients which prevent the growth of over a dozen strains of penicillin resistant bacteria and multiple strains of Staphylococcus.

The key to San Pedro's healing effect is the synergy between all of its medicinal alkaloids working collectively with one another under the guidance of the plants spirit or life-force. Yet the synergistic effect of San Pedro's ingredients does not just pertain to San Pedro alone, but rather pertains to all plant and power plant medicines. This is because single alkaloid pharmaceuticals and supplement extracts merely remove one part from the whole plant and then synthetically replicate that one ingredient so it can be patented and monopolized. Like most power plants in this chapter, San Pedro's consumption has been made illegal in most countries, so if you seek to work with the plant it is advised that you seek out a reputable center in a country where the medicine is legal for use and consumption.

"Plant based spirit guides, I do not call them drugs, if it's made by a human being in a laboratory it's a drug, if it's made by mother nature and is put on this planet to help us evolve, I take advantage of it."

-Terrence Mckenna

"Awareness is a primary component of consciousness and of individual potential and opportunity. Therefore, opening and expanding awareness by all means necessary may be considered the highest of human pursuits."

-Amazing Grace:
The Nine Principles of Living in Natural Magic

Coca Madre

While most people know that Cocaine is a toxic drug that certainly damages ones health, the actual Coca leaf which Cocaine is extracted and synthesized from is actually valued as a sacred medicine and super-food throughout numerous countries of South America. What makes Cocaine a harmful drug is the fact that it is only 1 of 14 medicinal alkaloids found in the Coca leaf, which only through heavy processing with synthetic chemicals such as kerosene and ammonia people are able to strip out of the plants leaves. In removing the cocaine alkaloid from the other 99.2% of ingredients comprising the coca leaf, the Cocaine then becomes toxic.

The Coca leaf in its unprocessed form is rich with numerous antioxidants as well as vitamins A, B1, B2 and C. Likewise the Coca leaf is rich in calcium, iron, phosphorus, riboflavin and protein. In a study conducted at Harvard University researchers found that chewing 100 grams of Coca leaves provided adults 100% of their daily nutritional requirements.

Aside from having a rich nutritional profile, Coca leaves also work as a healthy stimulant that accelerates mental concentration and energy similar to beverages such as coffee, green tea and yerba mate. In fact, in countries such as Peru, Bolivia and Ecuador, natives use Coca leaves as their preferred stimulant of choice. Coca leaf can be consumed by simply chewing the leaves, or through making a tea in hot water. Coca leaves are illegal to possess in most countries so be sure to consume coca leaves where they are legal.

MIND MUSHROOMS

Throughout history, ancient cultures living in North America, Europe, the Middle East and Central America have used specific psychoactive mushrooms such as Psilocybin and Amanita Muscaria varieties for healing and religious purposes. A modern day study conducted by Dr. Enzo Tagliazucci out of Germany's Goethe University revealed that the ingredients in these particular mushrooms work to alter consciousness in a specific way which can alleviate severe forms of depression and anxiety in those who properly consume them. MRI scans from Dr. Tagliazucci's study revealed that the Psilocybin mushroom activated areas of the brain involved in emotional thinking such as the hippocampus and anterior cingulate cortex and stimulates areas of the brain responsible for self-awareness and higher level thought processing.

In a similar study conducted at the University of Oxford, scientists studying the effects of Psilocybin mushrooms discovered that the mushroom worked to disconnect areas of the brain where depression and consciousness were linked, permitting one to experience states of hyper-awareness and feelings of oneness with the universe which lasted with them after the main experience of the mushrooms dissipated. Participants in this study reflected that they felt a dissolving of feelings relating to ego and selfishness and experienced deeper states of connectivity to all of their surroundings as well as inner peace. The Psilocybin and

Amanita Muscaria mushrooms are illegal in most countries and their use is not recommended where they are illegal.

"If the doors of perception were cleansed, every thing would appear to man as it is, infinite. For man has closed himself up, till he sees all things through narrow chinks of his cavern."

-William Blake

AETHEOGENS

As Entheogens work to invoke the Godliness and divinity of the mind, body and spirit, Aetheogens work to do the exact opposite in evoking the darker side of life, health and spirituality. An aethogenic substance is something derived via human processing and not through the self-organizing system of nature. Aethogenic substances work to distort our normal bodily functions and scramble as well as sometimes destroy our DNA codes which results in states of disharmony and dis-equalibrium which could be referred to as disease. Common Aetheogenic substances include pharmaceuticals, industrialized processed alcohols (beer, hard alcohol) and substances derived from petroleum such as plastics and synthetic chemicals. When introduced into the body these substances work to deplete our vital essences and overload our brains natural neurotransmitter balance which can often lead to permanent damage until Entheogens are introduced for healing and re-programming of our DNA. Aetheogens should be avoided by all means and safely tapered off of under the guidance of a qualified health practitioner.

Peyote

Peyote is a master plant that is not appropriate for most people as it is simply too strong and can be extremely frightening for those who are not well versed in Entheogens. The Peyote cactus has been used as a plant medicine by a vast majority of Native American tribes in the Southwestern United States and Central America for thousands of years where it is held as sacred. Peyote contains various alkaloids of which the primary one, like San Pedro, is Mescaline. While the San Pedro cactus also contains the Mescaline alkaloid, its concentration is significantly higher in Peyote and provides a stronger and different overall experience. The various alkaloids in Peyote have been shown to regulate neurotransmitters such as serotonin and dopamine as well as activate various neurotransmitter receptor sites and areas of the brain involving perception and cognition. Psychiatrist Dr. John Halpren's research on Peyote through the Native American Church revealed that similar to various other Entheogens, Peyote can be beneficial in the treatment of alcoholism and other drug addictions. Currently in America and most other countries the use of Peyote is illegal and restricted to be used only by those who are members of a Native America Church.

CANNABIS

Second only to that of the wild tobacco plant, the next greatest plant source of minerals on the planet can be found in that of Cannabis. While most of the public is under the impression that Cannabis's uses are limited merely to smoking the dry buds, the reality of the matter could not be further from the truth. While the smoking of Cannabis works to increase the potency of the plant's psychoactive chemical THC (Tetrahydrocannabinol) in a persons body, the greater medicinal benefits of the plant are completely bypassed in this manner, as the antioxidants and medicinal compounds found in the leaf and bud fail to be ingested by becoming destroyed by fire. When Cannabis is ingested raw however through the consumption of the plant's leaves, seeds, leaf juice or seed milk, the plants greater medicinal qualities become unlocked and available.

On top of containing an enormous storehouse of mind boosting minerals, the Cannabis leaves and buds when consumed in their raw state provide an abundance of antioxidants, anti-inflammatory compounds and specifically, a unique nutrient known as CBD (Cannabidiol). The compound CBD has been shown to enhance the neurotransmission capabilities of the brain and nervous system, providing enhanced synaptic communication and bioelectric conductivity to our neurogenic systems biologic matrix and integrative connectivity. While many corporate pharmaceutical companies are now trying to capitalize on the medicinal benefits of Marijuana through synthetically replicating the plants individual ingredients in order to obtain drug patents, these pharmaceutical replications are non-organic and lack the endless other medicinal ingredients found in the plant which support these compounds actions and benefits.

As well as the buds and leaves of the Cannabis plant, the plants seeds which are commonly referred to as hemp seeds, further contain numerous brain boosting benefits that support our overall health. On top of being a rich source of omega-3 and omega-6 fatty acids, hemp seeds further contain all 10 essential amino acids which make them a complete source of protein. Also found in hemp seeds are significant quantities of calcium, vitamin D, vitamin E, vitamin B12, phosphorous, magnesium and various other nutritive ingredients that support overall health.

Unlike hemp seeds which are legal everywhere for purchase, the rest of the Cannabis plant is only legal in certain parts of the world and therefore it is only recommended to consume the plant where it is legal and regulated. To get the raw benefits of Cannabis, look towards methods like blending, eating, juicing and salad making to extract the true un-tapped health benefits of this wonder herb.

NICOTIANA

One of the greatest sacred plants of all time which has been used ubiquitously throughout native cultures residing in both North and South America is that of wild tobacco. Unlike commercial cigarettes, pipe tobacco and chewing tobacco, which typically has over 4,000 synthetic chemicals added to it and is frequently found to contain less than 35% actual tobacco matter, wild tobacco is the greatest natural source of minerals found in any land plant on the planet and is also the most anti-parasitic plant yet discovered. Wild tobacco when eaten or juiced in proper quantities is shown to kill all parasites in their egg and larval stage, totally. Being that parasites and bad bacteria can work to hijack our physical energy and even our consciousness, drinking raw tobacco juice works as an invaluable tool to help us reclaim our energy levels through its dramatic cleansing abilities.

Little known to most regarding Tobacco's most prominent phytochemical Nicotine is that Nicotine is actually an antioxidant and B vitamin. A cousin of Niacin, which is vitamin B3, Nicotine or Nicotionic acid is actually a brain vitamin and has been shown to provide benefits to people suffering from Alzheimer's, Parkinson's, Schizophrenia and hyperactivity disorders. Specifically Nicotine is shown to work by switching on receptors in specific parts of the brain which activate the release of the neurotransmitter Dopamine. To get the benefits of Tobacco one can look towards smoke varieties such as organic or wild Nicotiana

Rustica, Mapacho, or other types of Native American heirloom varieties which have not been altered chemically or through genetic modification. These varieties need not be inhaled but rather puffed like a cigar, allowing for the beneficial plant phytochemicals to enter sublingually through the saliva. Tobacco juice is also a powerful health drink which can be consumed both through drinking and for those who dare, via enema applications.

PART IV
THE SPIRITUAL MIND

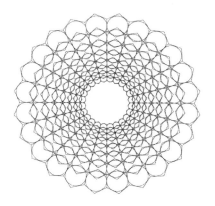

UNLOCK THE DOOR

"The inner world creates the outer world"

-David Wolfe

Before any great accomplishment can be brought into physical reality, it must first exist in the mind. At the foundation of achieving any accomplishment must lay a heartfelt belief and conviction that we can attain that which we seek. This involved absolute certainty and the elimination of all doubt. When one firmly decides that they deserve and have the power to attaining their goals, the doors of the universe immediately open up for them to step through, but first we must believe.

INTENTION

"Energy flows where attention goes"

-Makia

Before working to towards any goal it is imperative that one first sets their proper intention. Intentions that are fueled by love and one's mission contained in their heart are the only forms of intention retaining true cosmic powers to ascend one's spirit and bring about positive karma through positively contributing to the lives of others. Setting proper intention involves time for self-discovery and soul searching to reveal what lies beneath one's pre-conceived notions of what society tells them to think or become and finding in their true heart what their mission in life is.

KARMA

*"So whatever you wish that others would do to you,
do also to them, for this is the Law and the Prophets."*

-Matthew 7:12

Karma is the universes way of balancing and self-regulating
the free will of every cosmic soul. The prime rule of karma
is that every action one takes whether positive or negative
will result in the exact same positive or negative action
returning to the person whether in this present incarnation
or in a future incarnation. To bring about good karma for
yourself and others it is necessary to practice the golden
rule. Practicing the golden rule ensures that you are casting
out positive and loved filled actions in your life and will
return to you in the forms of joy, abundance, peace and
other unimaginable forms of positive circumstances.

Vision Quest

The mind is a tool which can be used to fulfill our higher purpose in life, or be a ship left unattended without a captain. In getting the most from our mind we must steer it in the direction of our own goals and not those of someone else. Through writing down our goals we are able to see our dreams on paper and further instill them into our consciousness through the window of our eyes. See your goals through this window and take massive *action* to push towards them through all obstacles. A noble captain of the mind can only be found in the heart, which entails opening up the heart chakra energy to states of love and letting go of fear which manifests as low vibrational energy and stagnation. If the heart is not in control of the mind than the mind will take over and override one's consciousness with endless un-productive thoughts. These thoughts are actually distractions and a leech of ones vital energies. Find what makes your heart sing and steer the ship of your mind in the direction of your higher mission in life, without fears of how your actions may unfold in the future.

> *"Every great work, every big accomplishment, has been brought into manifestation through holding to the vision, and often just before the big achievement, comes apparent failure and discouragement."*
>
> -Florence Scoval Shinn

THAT WHICH WE CONSUME

"It's called tell, a, vision, programming."

-Eddie Griffin

In our daily lives we consume not only the food we put in our mouths, but also that which we take in through our eyes, ears, physical sensations and the mind. When we view TV shows, images and news filled with fear, violence or materialism, we put ourselves at risk of taking these toxic messages away with us. Such things can steer us in the wrong direction from that which we truly seek in life. Be mindful of the things you take in through your senses, and make sure they work to uplift you and not lead you astray. Seek to consume information that supports your physical and mental health as well as spiritual growth. If what we consume becomes a part of us then this area should be given the utmost attentiveness and personal discipline.

AVENUES OF CONSUMPTION

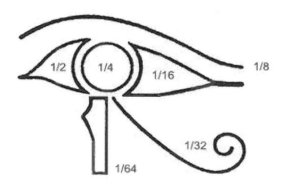

*

1/2 = Smell

    1/4 = Sight

        1/8 = Thought

            1/16 = Hearing

                1/32 = Taste

                    1/64 = Touch

                        * = Intuitive Feeling

Understanding What's Real

"Where there is perception, there is deception"

—Buddha

That which we perceive is often not what is reality. The mind has a way of seeing what it wants and even more so, what it fears. In fine-tuning our minds we must always be aware of their great artistic abilities to script illusions which are not real. In dealing with our minds perceptions it is best not to repress them but to step back as a third party and acknowledge them. Ask yourself: Why do I have these thoughts? Is there some experience from my past which has led me to this pre-conception? In stepping back and witnessing our thoughts as a neutral bystander, we can make our false perceptions powerless and work to strengthen our open mindedness and higher awareness instead.

High Vibrational Frequencies

In studies conducted by molecular biologist Dr. Glen Rein, samples of placenta were administered to people who emitted both extreme feelings of anger and extreme feelings of love at the tissue samples. The placenta that received emotional energies of anger reacted by having it's DNA damaged and eventually uncoiled and destroyed. In turn however, when these destroyed samples were then given to people whom evoked feelings of extreme love onto the placenta, their DNA structure was witnessed to completely re-organize their structure and heal. These experiments work to reveal how the power of love can be just as healing as the power of fear can be damaging to biologic life. Feelings of love in this experiment were evidenced as having the ability to physically open up ones DNA phantom so that this DNA could physically absorb photons of light/energy. The power of loves vibrational energy can be administered to you by your own self and transmitted to others to help them receive healing benefits in turn. Likewise, the act of praying over ones food in thankfulness and gratitude before eating has been shown to have energetic effects on the food which energetically change its vibration when electrically monitored. Best of all is that giving love and gratitude is free.

Social Relationships

Throughout 98% of human history people have lived indigenously in self-supporting abundant communities of a tribal nature. In these communities people support one another in all walks of life and any detriment or gain to one is considered a detriment or gain to all. As a result of the birth of capitalism and economic based agricultural societies however, this communal based lifestyle has become inverted, giving rise to the illusion of separateness and the mindset that one must only work for the greater good of themself, neglecting the abundance of others. This mindset can cause people to lack fulfilling social relationships with others and live more isolated lifestyles which further perpetuates personal feelings of separateness and isolation. Lacking social relationships is not only a lonely form of existence but typically leads to greater experiences of depression, anxiety and feelings of disconnection from the greater universe and nature. Seeking out meaningful relationships in your life which support your personal growth and evolution, while releasing fears a pre-conceived notions of competition can help one in all aspects of their daily lives. In seeking out social relationships, look for others who you find inspiring, knowledgeable and kind hearted. Friends who have your best intentions as an equal priority with their own will not only help you grow mentally and spiritually, but will also create new paths for joy and unique life experiences that are available at every moment.

THE PHARMACEUTICAL TRAP

In an effort to deal with the hardships that life presents us in our current western society, many have been coerced into taking synthetically produced, mind altering pharmaceuticals to help cope with life's un-pleasantries. Unfortunately, when these methods are taken they not only cause damage to the brain's natural biology and synchronicity, but also can frequently work to divert one off of their true path in life through numbing one's mind and intuition. Antidepressants containing fluoride or fluorine are the absolute worst of these culprits as these synthetic chemicals specifically latch on to one's pineal gland which is the spiritual center of the mind and can cause one to become disassociated from their higher self, true life mission and forming deeper relationships with others. Implementing the variety of steps in this book will work in an integrated manner to help one improve their mental harmony and detoxification of harmful chemicals. In regards to circumstances of depression and anxiety, this author's personal opinion is that this is best addressed with the medicine of Ayahuasca in a location where it is legal and one can be medically assessed and guided by a trained health practitioner.

Spelling, Words and Spell-Casting

We have come to a point in time where we as a global civilization have lost our once held wisdom regarding the power of words, names, writing and language. Words and phrases, regardless of what language they are in, contain within them a vibrational code which when spoken or written transmutes their information and meaning out into the greater cosmos as a spell to be manifested. Whether the manifestation occurs immediately or at a future point in time is out of one's control, but what is in one's control are the names, words and even thoughts which they choose in their daily lives. To tap into the power of The Word, write down your goals on paper as if they are already manifested and alive. Statements such as "I am the greatest... ever" taps into the infinite possibilities of self-manifestation which we all have access to at any time. Be conscious of the names you take on or which may have been spell-cast onto you and research each syllables definition. These syllables or words frequently stem from Latin or other historic languages so be mindful of this fact. Ask yourself, does the definition of this word or name suite your goals and aspirations in life? If not, through the power of free will you can consciously choose at any point in time to re-write your destiny, on your own terms.

THE ART OF LETTING GO

The feeling that one needs to have control over every unfolding outcome in their life is quite pervasive in our world today. Yet life never manifests exactly as we try to paint it. There appears to be guiding forces beyond our total comprehension which exist, routing our life's course like a flowing stream guides water from a spring to the ocean. To tap into this natural flow and allow for your life's mission to manifest as it is meant to, one must learn the art of surrender. This is the art of letting go of trying to control the future and merely doing what your heart tells you is right to do at the present moment in your life. This involves self-discovery and soul-searching to unveil what you are truly meant to be doing here in this life incarnation. With surrender comes true freedom and enlightenment. You can finally relax.

"The past is history (his-story), the future is a mystery (mis-story) and the present is a gift we give ourselves today."

Sacred Geometry

Ancient geometric images such as "The Flower of Life" symbol have been found carved into countless religious and sacred sites throughout the world such as the Egyptian Pyramids, The Sacred Valley of Peru, The Mesada in Israel and countless other locations. In studying the history of these various sacred geometric symbols, a story is revealed showing that contained in their structure lies specific blueprints containing the fabric and make-up of our organic universe on a holographic and multidimensional level. Shapes such as the Flower of Life, The Seed of Life, the Vesica Pices, Metatron's Cube and various others, when taken in through the eyes and, or drawn by hand have the potential to activate specific changes both genetically in our DNA, as well as in our energetic chakra system that can help us to activate higher potentials of intelligence, creativity and perception. Various teachings on Sacred Geometry exist on the internet and in books. Peer into them and see where you're led.

The Law of Harmony

"Ultimately, man should not ask what the meaning of his life is, but rather he must recognize that it is he who is asked."

-Viktor E. Frankl

When we are born, our minds are perfect and contain all the potential necessary to achieve that which we seek. Although the positive and negative experiences we encounter in life may trick us into thinking our potential is limited, at the foundation of the mind lays perfection. In the heart of this perfection exist the two dueling forces of love and fear. If we allow our imaginations fears to get the best of our mind, then we can unknowingly attract the very things we wished to avoid. That is why in mastering the mind and overcoming the obstacle of fear, the best remedy is to take bold action and cultivate our true core's spirit of unconditional love. For the only way we can ever achieve in life is through either our love for ourselves, or our love for an-other. If fear drives us to thinking that the only way to win in life is if another fails, then we have already failed. Yet when we instill our minds to take on a win-win mindset and appreciate the oneness of all things in our planet and the universe, we unlock the final doors to infinite intelligence, and allow the true perfection of our minds to begin to emerge.

CONCLUSION

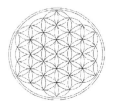

It is my hope that you may manifest acts of unconditional love towards yourself and towards others. Love yourself by eating only the purest healthiest foods, drinking only the most vibrant flowing natural spring water, breathing the most life filled fresh air, basking in the suns light and allowing your body to run freely through the countless forms of motion and exercise we have discovered as man. Think deeply as to what it is you seek in life and write down exactly how you will achieve your dreams. As you strengthen your mind through improving it physically and spiritually, bridge the gap between the intentions of your goals and the power of your intelligence. Unite the two for the common good of yourself and your fellow friends on this planet. Remember, that

at the heart of the universe has always been love and benevolence. It can be found in the suns shining light which provides warmth for our bodies and food for the plants which give us oxygen. It can be found in the endless colorful fruit trees which decorate our planet and provide us food freely. It can be found through the springs of pure water which flow life into forests, mountains and rivers for all things to drink. And it can be found at the inception of life in a mothers natural instinct to feed her newborn child through the giving of her own milk, just as her mother Earth did for her. What we see in life is just a reflection of our inner state of mind. Recognize the beauty in life and you will forever shine.

Appendix A: Living Spring Water

All spring water is not created equal. You may be surprised to learn that nearly all of the bottled spring water you find at your supermarket is either not spring water at all, or is spring water that has been processed through ozonation, UV exposure and dilution with tap water. The reason for this is because lobbyists have pushed for corporations to be able to label their water as "spring water" even if it is actually well water. Furthermore the law has allowed for bottled spring water companies to dilute their water with up to 50% tap water which is to say the least, not so appetizing. If you are one of the few people to find real bottled spring water in a store, while the water may truly be from a spring, it has most likely been ozonated to kill off any living properties in the water. This destroys the living properties makes spring water so valuable. To avoid all of this confusion and deception you can simply get your water for free by going to real springs, just as people have always done throughout history.

*Utilize the free online database www.findaspring.com and find a spring near you.

Appendix B: Sun Tips

While the sun is a major provider of life and health, certain modern technologies will counteract the healing effects of the sun, and can reverse them from healthful to harmful. The healthy UVB rays of the sun cannot penetrate glass and sunlight transmitted through glass onto the skin will promote burning rather than health. As well, the Vitamin D our bodies produce as a result of sunlight is maintained in our bodies natural oils. Therefore, using soap within a 48 hour period of receiving sun can actually wash away these vitamin D containing oils and prevent us from absorbing the Vitamin D into our bloodstreams. My personal stance on sunscreen is that it is a dangerous product due to the synthetic chemicals used in most lotions. Sunscreen can also work to block UVB light from penetrating the skin and the chemicals in the lotion can be ingested into our bodies through the pores on our skin. To best protect yourself from sun overexposure I recommend loading up on antioxidant rich foods prior to sun exposure such as green tea, berries and other nutrient rich organic fruits and vegetables. If you have circumstances which require you to spend unusually long hours in the sun, or you burn easily, consider using a protective hat or seek out a sunscreen lotion that is certified organic as these are much safer alternatives to standard commercial sunscreens.

APPENDIX C: CRACKING OPEN
THE PINEAL GLAND

In order for us to tap into our deepest states of intuition, intelligence and spiritual enlightenment is necessary to unlock and activate our brains Pineal Gland. Commonly referred to by ancient cultures, and mystics as, "the third eye," our pineal gland sits in the center of our brain between our right and left hemispheres and is responsible for producing neurotransmitters such as serotonin and melatonin. Yet the pineal gland wasn't bestowed the name "third eye" for just any random reason. Rather, when dissected from the brain it is found that the pineal gland actually contains photoreceptors just like our own two seeing eyes and is actually activated by light transmitted through our two eyes which works to stimulate the pineal gland. This sunlight transmitted through our eyes stimulates the pineal glands production of serotonin and further works to strengthen the gland's ability to break free of specific harmful chemicals that can encrust it. As well, the pineal gland is also stimulated by darkness in which the gland responds by producing melatonin to help induce us into sleep.

Sun -> Serotonin

Moon -> Melatonin

As a result of our natural biological make up, the pineal gland although part of the brain, is not protected by the blood brain barrier and therefore does not have an extra line of defense against harmful toxins that enter the bloodstream. Specific toxins such as synthetic fluoride and synthetic calcium are specifically shown to have an affinity for the pineal gland and in which case they coat and encrust it, weakening the glands abilities to produce our neurotransmitters and receive photons of light from the sun, moon and stars. Yet it is important to distinguish the difference between synthetic fluoride and synthetic calcium versus organic fluoride and organic calcium. If received from plant sources such as vegetables and other organic foods, calcium and fluoride are healthy essential minerals. Yet when fluoride and calcium are synthetically manufactured through industrial processing and added to tap water, vitamin supplements, toothpastes, fortified cereals and various other products, these synthetic minerals are shown to have detrimental affects to the pineal gland as well as numerous other organs of the body.

Before beginning to activate ones pineal gland it is to necessary to remove the toxic chemicals that prevent it from working such as synthetic fluoride, synthetic calcium, pharmaceutical medications and other toxins as mentioned above. If you are drinking tap water then look to replace this with purer and safer options such as natural spring water, well water, reverse osmosis water, or carbon-filtered water. From there, one can work to remove any vitamin supplements, mineral fortified foods and toothpastes containing added fluoride or calcium. Last but not least, one can take five minutes out of their day to install a carbon shower filter which works to remove chlorine, fluoride, used toilet paper particles and other impurities from tap water that can enter our bodies through the skin, pores and lungs when we shower.

After one has begun removing the impurities that prevent the pineal gland from being activated they can start implementing practices that work to stimulate and grow their pineal gland's functioning and abilities. A great practice that one can do throughout their life is that of meditating. The act of meditating works to stimulate the chakra system of our brain and body that's responsible for conducting and generating life-force energy. Meditating specifically guides bioelectric and zero-point energy to the pineal gland allowing for greater states of clarity and intuition to come into our conscious life.

Following meditation, a more advanced exercise modality which works to activate the pineal gland as well as all of the body's chakra points is that of Kundalini Yoga. The Kundalini which rests coiled in the lowest chakra of our spine is a transducer of energy which rises farther up the spine through the practice until finally reaching the pineal gland/third eye chakra. Upon activating the Kundalini and growing its pathway to the pineal gland, one is able to merge the photon celestial energy of the sun and cosmos with that of the physical body which roots to the Earth. Being that the bones of our skeletal system are technically piezoelectric crystals at the core, the Kundalini energy rises and flows through the crystal bones of the spine, activating the 33 vertebrae points one by one until reaching the crown and pineal gland energy points at the top levels of the upper spine.

In the food category numerous options are available for accelerating and detoxifying our brain's pineal gland. As a foundation one should look to comprise the percentage of foods in their diet to a highest degree of organic plants and animals as possible. Eating organic adds a buffer to protect oneself from pesticides, herbicides, fungicides, GMO's and other harmful chemical laden substances that can wreak havoc on our mental and physical health. Foods that specifically support and activate the pineal gland are tumeric (tea and raw), cacao beans, green plants and vegetables, wild harvested spring water, reishi mushroom tea, grass juices, beets, apple cider vinegar and others. Supplements one can use to help detoxify and activate the pineal gland are zeolite tinctures, bentonite clay, organic MSM powder and ormus gold. Begin activating your pineal gland today and tap into levels of your higher self that lay dormant, calling to be awakened.

Visit Joshua Eagle at:

www.joshuaeagle.com

www.bloominati.com

BIBLIOGRAPHY:

Adams JB, Audhya T, McDonough-Means S, Rubin RA, Quig D, Geis E, Gehn E, Loresto M, Mitchell J, Atwood S, Barnhouse S, Lee W. Toxicological status of children with autism vs. neurotypical children and the association with autism severity. Biological Trace Element Research. 2013 Feb;151(2):171-80.

Aguirre Moreno AC, Campos Peña V, Villeda Hernández J, León Rivera I, Montiel Arcos E. Ganoderma lucidum reduces kainic acid-induced hippocampal neuronal damage via inflammatory cytokines and glial fibrillary acid protein expression. Proceedings of the Western Pharmacology Society. 2011;54:78-9.

Amanda J. Jenkins, Teobaldo Llosa, Ivan Montoya, and Edward J. Cone. Identification and quantitation of alkaloids in coca tea. Forensic Sci Int. Feb 9, 1996; 77(3): 179–189.

Annweiler C, Allali G, Allain P, Bridenbaugh S, Schott AM, Kressig RW, Beauchet O. Vitamin D and cognitive performance in adults: a systematic review. Eur J Neurol. 2009 Oct;16(10):1083-9.

Arora, D. Mushrooms demystified, 2nd edition. Ten Speed Press. (1986).

Aschoff, J., 'Annual Rhythms in Man', in Aschoff, J. (ed.), Handbook of Behavioural Neurobiology, Plenum Press, New York, 1981.

Assunção M, Santos-Marques MJ, Carvalho F, Andrade JP. Green tea averts age-dependent decline of hippocampal signaling systems related to antioxidant defenses and survival. Free Radical Biology and Medicine. 2010 Mar 15;48(6):831-8.

Balion C, Griffith LE, Strifler L, Henderson M, Patterson C, Heckman G, Llewellyn DJ, Raina P. Vitamin D, cognition, and dementia: a systematic review and meta-analysis. Neurology. 2012 Sep 25;79(13):1397-405.

Baroni L, Scoglio S, Benedetti S, Bonetto C, Pagliarani S, Benedetti Y, Rocchi M, Canestrari F. Effect of a Klamath algae product ("AFA-B12⊠) on blood levels of vitamin B12 and homocysteine in vegan subjects: a pilot study. Int J Vitam Nutr Res. 2009 Mar;79(2):117-23. doi: 10.1024/0300-9831.79.2.117.

Benedetti S, Benvenuti F, Pagliarani S, Francogli S, Scoglio S, Canestrari F. Antioxidant properties of a novel phycocyanin extract from the blue-green alga Aphanizomenon flos-aquae. Life Sci. 2004 Sep 24;75(19):2353-62.

Benedetti S, Benvenuti F, Scoglio S, Canestrari F. Oxygen radical absorbance capacity of phycocyanin and phycocyanobilin from the food supplement Aphanizomenon flos-aquae. J Med Food. 2010 Feb;13(1):223-7. doi: 10.1089/jmf.2008.0257.

Beom Jae Lee and Young-Tae Bak. "Irritable Bowel Syndrome, Gut Microbiota and Probiotics". J Neurogastroenterol Motil. 2011 July; 17(3): 252–266. Published online 2011 July 13.

Bercik P, Park AJ, Sinclair D, Khoshdel A, Lu J, Huang X, Deng Y, Blennerhassett PA, Fahnestock M, Moine D, Berger B, Huizinga JD, Kunze W, McLean PG, Bergonzelli GE, Collins SM, Verdu EF. "The anxiolytic effect of Bifidobacterium longum NCC3001 involves vagal pathways for gut-brain communication. Neurogastroenterol Motil. 2011 Dec;23(12):1132-9.

Bercik, P. et al.; Chronic Gastrointestinal Inflammation Induces Anxiety-Like Behavior and Alters Central Nervous System Biochemistry in Mice. Gastroenterology. Vol 139 : 6, 2102-2112.e1, Dec 2010.

Berg JM, Tymoczko JL, Stryer L. Biochemistry. 5th edition. New York: W H Freeman; 2002. Section 30.2, Each Organ Has a Unique Metabolic Profile.

Bibliography:

Bravo JA, Forsythe P, Chew MV, Escaravage E, Savignac HM, Dinan TG, Bienenstock J, Cryan JF. Ingestion of Lactobacillus strain regulates emotional behavior and central GABA receptor expression in a mouse via the vagus nerve. Proc Natl Acad Sci U S A. 2011 Sep 20;108(38):16050-5.

Buys YM, Alasbali T, Jin YP, Smith M, Gouws P, Geffen N, Flanagan JG, Shapiro CM, Trope GE. Effect of sleeping in a head-up position on intraocular pressure in patients with glaucoma. Ophthalmology. 2010 Jul;117(7):1348-51.

Bytingsvik J, Lie E, Aars J, Derocher AE, Wiig Ø, Jenssen BM. PCBs and OH-PCBs in polar bear mother-cub pairs:

a comparative study based on plasma levels in 1998 and 2008. Sci Total Environ. 2012 Feb 15;417-418:117-28.

C. Borek. "Antioxidant Health Effects of Aged Garlic Extract," Journal of Nutrition, vol. 131, no. 3, pp. 1010S–1015S, 2001.

C.A. Lowrya, J.H. Hollisa, A. de Vriesa, B. Pana, L.R. Brunetb, J.R.F. Huntb, J.F.R. Patonc, E. van Kampena, D.M. Knighta, A.K. Evansa, G.A.W. Rookb and S.L. Lightmana. Identification of an immune-responsive meso-limbocortical serotonergic system: Potential role in regulation of emotional behavior." Neuroscience. 2007 March 28.

C.C. Streeter, P.L. Gerbarg, R.B. Saper, D.A. Ciraulo, R.P. Brown. Effects of yoga on the autonomic nervous system, gamma-aminobutyric-acid, and allostasis in epilepsy, depression, and post-traumatic stress disorder. Medical Hypotheses. Volume 78, Issue 5 , Pages 571-579, May 2012

Carhart-Harris RL1, Erritzoe D, Williams T, Stone JM, Reed LJ, Colasanti A, Tyacke RJ, Leech R, Malizia AL, Murphy K, Hobden P, Evans J, Feilding A, Wise RG, Nutt DJ. Neural correlates of the psychedelic state as determined by fMRI studies with psilocybin. Natl Acad Sci U S A. 2012 Feb 7;109(6):2138-43. doi: 10.1073/pnas.1119598109. Epub 2012 Jan 23.

Carmia Borek. Garlic Reduces Dementia and Heart-Disease Risk.

Cavendish R, ed. (1994). Man, Myth and Magic - Volume 19. New York, NY: Marshall Cavendish.

Chevalier G, Sinatra ST, Oschman JL, Sokal K, Sokal P. Earthing: health implications of reconnecting the human body to the Earth's surface electrons. J Environ Public Health. 2012;2012:291541.

Chu SF, Zhang JT. New achievements in ginseng research and its future prospects. Chinese Journal of Integrative Medicine. 2009 Dec;15(6):403-8.

Chung S. Yang, Saranjit K. Chhabra, Jun-Yan Hong and Theresa J. SmitMechanisms of Inhibition of Chemical Toxicity and Carcinogenesis by Diallyl Sulfide (DAS) and Related Compounds from Garlic. Laboratory for Cancer Research, College of Pharmacy, Rutgers, The State University of New Jersey, Piscataway, NJ 08854-8020

Cranson, R. W.; et al. "Transcendental Meditation and Improved Performance on Intelligence Related Measures: A Longitudinal Study." Personality and Individual Differences 12 (1991): 1105-1116.

Creer DJ, Romberg C, Saksida LM, van Praag H, Bussey TJ. Running enhances spatial pattern separation in mice. Proceedings of The National Academy of Sciences of The United States of America. 2010 Feb 2;107(5):2367-72.

Cryan JF, Dinan TG. Mind-altering microorganisms: the impact of the gut microbiota on brain and behaviour. Nature Reviews. Neuroscience. 2012 Oct;13(10):701-12.

D'Angelo L, Grimaldi R, Caravaggi M, Marcoli M, Perucca E, Lecchini S, Frigo GM, Crema A. A double-blind, placebo-controlled clinical study on the effect of a standardized ginseng extract on psychomotor performance in healthy volunteers. Journal of Ethnopharmacology. 1986 Apr-May;16(1):15-22.

Darbinyan V, Aslanyan G, Amroyan E, Gabrielyan E, Malmström C, Panossian A (2007). "Clinical trial of Rhodiola rosea L. extract in the treatment of mild to moderate depression". Nord J Psychiatry 61 (5): 343–8.

Darbinyan V, Kteyan A, Panossian A, Gabrielian E, Wikman G, Wagner H (Oct 2000). "Rhodiola rosea in stress induced fatigue—a double blind cross-over study of a standardized extract with a repeated low-dose regimen on the mental performance of healthy physicians during night duty". Phytomedicine 7 (5): 365–71.

Das A, Banik NL, Ray SK. Garlic compounds generate reactive oxygen species leading to activation of stress kinases and cysteine proteases for apoptosis in human glioblastoma T98G and U87MG cells. Cancer. 2007 Sep 1;110(5):1083-95.

De Paulis, Tomas; Martin, Peter R (April 27, 2004). "Cerebral effects of noncaffeine constituents in roasted coffee". In Nehlig, Astrid. Coffee, Tea, Chocolate, and the Brain. London: Taylor & Francis. pp. 187–196. ISBN 0-415-30691-4.

De Vendômois JS, Roullier F, Cellier D, Séralini GE. A

Comparison of the Effects of Three GM Corn Varieties on Mammalian Health. Int J Biol Sci 2009; 5(7):706-726.

Department of Public Health and Family Medicine, Tufts University School of Medicine, Boston, MA 02111

Di X, Yan J, Zhao Y, Zhang J, Shi Z, Chang Y, Zhao B. L-theanine protects the APP (Swedish mutation) transgenic SH-SY5Y cell against glutamate-induced excitotoxicity via inhibition of the NMDA receptor pathway.Neuroscience. 2010 Jul 14;168(3):778-86.

Duncko R, Cornwell B, Cui L, Merikangas KR, Grillon C.Acute exposure to stress improves performance in trace eyeblink conditioning and spatial learning tasks in healthy men. Learning & Memory. 2007 May 1;14(5):329-35.

Dwyer AV, Whitten DL, Hawrelak JA (March 2011)."Herbal medicines, other than St. John's Wort, in the treatment of depression: a systematic review" (PDF).Altern Med Rev 16 (1): 40–9. PMID 21438645.

Erickson KI, Voss MW, Prakash RS, Basak C, Szabo A, Chaddock L, Kim JS, Heo S, Alves H, White SM, Wojcicki TR, Mailey E,Vieira VJ, Martin SA, Pence BD, Woods JA, McAuley E, Kramer AF. Exercise training increases size of hippocampus and improves memory.

Erowid. (2002): Mucuna pruriens. Created 2002-APR-22. Retrieved 2007-DEC-17.

Eser O, Songur A, Yaman M, Cosar M, Fidan H, Sahin O, Mollaoglu H, Buyukbas S. The protective effect of avocado soybean unsaponifilables on brain ischemia/reperfusion injury in rat prefrontal cortex. British Journal of Neurosurgery. 2011 Dec;25(6):701-6.

Eskelinen MH, Kivipelto M. Caffeine as a protective factor in dementia and Alzheimer's disease. J Alzheimers Dis. 2010;20 Suppl 1:S167-74. doi: 10.3233/JAD-2010-1404.

Fossati, C. "On the virtue and therapeutic properties of 'yerba-maté' (Ilex paraguayensis or paraguariensis St. Hilaire 1838)." Clin. Ter. 1976; 78(3): 265–72.

G. Oboh, et al.; "Food Chemistry"; Hot pepper (Capsicum Annuum, Tepin and Capsicum Chinese, Habanero) Prevents Fe2+-Induced Lipid Peroxidation in Brain -- In Vitro; 2007.

G. Oboh, et al.; "Journal of Medicinal Food"; Hot Pepper (Capsicum spp.) Protects Brain from Sodium Nitroprusside- and Quinolinic Acid-Induced Oxidative Stress In Vitro; July 2008.

Ganiyu Oboh, et al.;"Experimental and Toxicologic Pathology"; Cyclophosphamide-Induced Oxidative Stress in Brain: Protective Effect of Hot Short Pepper (Capsicum Frutescens L. Var. Abbreviatum); May 2010

Ganpat TS, Nagendra HR. Yoga therapy for developing emotional intelligence in mid-life managers. Journal of Midlife Health. 2011 Jan;2(1):28-30.

Gao L, Fang JS, Bai XY, Zhou D, Wang YT, Liu AL, Du GH. In silico target fishing for the potential targets and molecular mechanisms of baicalein as an anti-parkinsonian agent: discovery of the protective effects on NMDA receptor-mediated neurotoxicity. Chemical Biology and Drug Design. 2013 Mar 5.

Garner SC, Mar MH, Zeisel SH. Choline distribution and metabolism in pregnant rats and fetuses are influenced by the choline content of the maternal diet. The Journal of Nutrition. 1995 Nov;125(11):2851-8.-Meck WH, Williams CL. Characterization of the facilitative effects of perinatal choline supplementation on timing and temporal memory. Neuroreport. 1997 Sep 8;8(13):2831-5.

Gen X/Y Moms Study, Produce for Better Health Foundation, March 2011.

Ghaly M, Teplitz D. The biologic effects of grounding the human body during sleep as measured by cortisol levels and subjective reporting of sleep, pain, and stress. Journal of Alternative and Complementary Medicine. 2004 Oct;10(5):767-76.

Gilroy DJ, Kauffman KW, Hall RA, Huang X, Chu FS. Assessing potential health risks from microcystin toxins in blue-green algae dietary supplements. Environ Health Perspect. 2000 May;108(5):435-9.

Grant WB. Does vitamin D reduce the risk of dementia? J Alzheimers Dis. 2009;17(1):151-9.

Ha Z, Zhu Y, Zhang X, et al. (Sep 2002). "[The effect of rhodiola and acetazolamide on the sleep architecture and blood oxygen saturation in men living at high altitude]" (in Chinese). Zhonghua Jie He He Hu Xi Za Zhi 25 (9): 527–30. PMID 12423559.

Hadhazy, A. "Think Twice : How the Gut's "Second Brain" Influences Mood and Well Being". Scientific American, February 12, 2010.

Haider S, Batool Z, Tabassum S, Perveen T, Saleem S, Naqvi F, Javed H, Haleem DJ. Effects of walnuts (Juglans regia) on learning and memory functions. Plant Foods For Human Nutrition. 2011 Nov;66(4):335-40.

Hashimoto M, Kanda M, Ikeno K, Hayashi Y, Nakamura T, Ogawa Y, Fukumitsu H, Nomoto H, Furukawa S. Oral administration of royal jelly facilitates mRNA expression of glial cell line-derived neurotrophic factor and neurofilament H in the hippocampus of the adult mouse brain. Bioscience, Biotechnology, and Biochemistry. 2005 Apr;69(4):800-5.

Hattori N, Nomoto H, Fukumitsu H, Mishima S, Furukawa S. Royal jelly and its unique fatty acid, 10-hydroxy-trans-2-decenoic acid, promote neurogenesis byneural stem/progenitor cells in vitro. Biomedical Research. 2007 Oct;28(5):261-6.

Hattori N, Ohta S, Sakamoto T, Mishima S, Furukawa S. Royal jelly facilitates restoration of the cognitive ability in trimethyltin-intoxicated mice. Evidence Based Complementary and Alternative Medicine. 2011;2011:165968. doi: 10.1093/ecam/nep029. Epub 2010 Oct 25.

Higdon, Jane; Linus Pauling Institute; Essential Fatty Acids; December 2005

Ho YS, Yu MS, Yang XF, So KF, Yuen WH, Chang RC. Neuroprotective effects of polysaccharides from wolfberry, the fruits of Lycium barbarum, against homocysteine-induced toxicity in rat cortical neurons. Journal of Alzheimers Disease. 2010;19(3):813-27.

Hollis B.W. Circulating 25-hydroxyvitamin D levels indicative of vitamin D sufficiency: implications for establishing a new effective dietary intake recommendation for vitamin D". Journal of Nutrition. 2005 Feb;135(2):317-22.

Hölzel BK, Carmody J, Vangel M, Congleton C, Yerramsetti SM, Gard T, Lazar SW. Mindfulness practice leads to increases in regional brain gray matter density. Psychiatry Res. 2011 Jan 30;191(1):36-43. doi: 10.1016/j.pscychresns.2010.08.006. Epub 2010 Nov 10.

Horne B, et al; Intermountain Medical Center (2011, May 20). Routine periodic fasting is good for your health, and your heart, study suggests. ScienceDaily.

http://biopark.org/peru/Huachuma-healing.html

http://en.wikipedia.org/wiki/Coca

http://www.epa.gov/opptintr/pubs/chemmgmt/products.pdf

http://www.ewg.org/research/
body-burden-pollution-newborns

http://www.naturalnews.com/036650_synthetic_vitamins_disease_side_effects.html

http://www.power-of-turmeric.com/curcumin-and-brain-health.html

Javier A. Bravo, Paul Forsythe, Marianne V. Chew, Emily Escaravage, Hélène M. Savignac, Timothy G. Dinan, John Bienenstock, John F. Cryan. Ingestion of Lactobacillus strain regulates emotional behavior and central GABA receptor expression in a mouse via the vagus nerve.Proceedings of the National Academy of Sciences, 2011; DOI: 10.1073/pnas.1102999108

Jenks S, Matthews D. "Ingestion of Mycobacterium vaccae influences learning and anxiety in mice." Presented at the Annual Animal Behavior Society Meeting, William and Mary College, Williamsburg, VA July 25 – 30, 2010.

Jones, Kenneth (1990), Reishi: Ancient Herb for Modern Times, Sylvan Press, p. 6.

K. M. Neufeld, N. Kang, J. Bienenstock, J. A. Foster. Reduced anxiety-like behavior and central neurochemical change in germ-free mice. Neurogastroenterology & Motility

Katzenschlager, R, et al;. (2004): Mucuna pruriens in Parkinson's disease: a double blind clinical and pharmacological study. Journal of Neurology Neurosurgery and Psychiatry75(12): 1672–1677.

Kay RA. Microalgae as food and supplement. Crit Rev Food Sci Nutr. 1991;30(6):555-73. Review.

Kelsey N, Hulick W, Winter A, Ross E, Linseman D.Neuroprotective effects of anthocyanins on apoptosis induced by mitochondrial oxidative stress. Nutritional Neuroscience. 2011 Nov;14(6):249-59.

Kennedy DO, Scholey AB, Wesnes KA. Modulation of cognition and mood following administration of single doses of Ginkgo biloba, ginseng, and a ginkgo/ginseng combination to healthy young adults. Physiology & Behavior. 2002 Apr 15;75(5):739-51.

King James Bible (Cambridge Ed.)

Kjeld T, Pott FC, Secher NH. Facial immersion in cold water enhances cerebral blood velocity during breath-hold exercise in humans. Journal of Applied Physiology. 2009 Apr;106(4):1243-8.

Klark, K. University of Kansas Press Release; More Proof That Green Tea May Postpone Cancer, Heart Disease; September 1997

Krikorian R, Shidler MD, Nash TA, Kalt W, Vinqvist-Tymchuk MR, Shukitt-Hale B, Joseph JA. Blueberry supplementation improves memory in older adults. J Agric Food Chem. 2010 Apr 14;58(7):3996-4000.

Kulshreshtha A et al. "Current Pharmaceutical Biotechnology"; Spirulina in Health Care Management; Oct 2008.

L. Zhang, et. al., "Exogenous plant MIR168a specifically targets mammalian LDLRAP1: evidence of cross-kingdom regulation by microRNA," Cell Research, doi:10.1038/cr.2011.158, 2011.

Lin SM, Wang SW, Ho SC, Tang YL. Protective effect of green tea -epigallocatechin-3-gallate against the monoamine oxidase B enzyme activity increase in adult rat brains. Nutrition. 2010 Nov-Dec;26(11-12):1195-200. doi: 10.1016/j.nut.2009.11.022. Epub 2010 May 15.

Liu Q, Liu ZL, Tian X (Feb 2008). "[Phenolic components from Rhodiola dumulosa]" (in Chinese).Zhongguo Zhong Yao Za Zhi 33 (4): 411–3.PMID 18533499.

Lublin A, Isoda F, Patel H, Yen K, Nguyen L, Hajje D, Schwartz M, Mobbs C. FDA-approved drugs that protect mammalian neurons from glucose toxicity slow aging dependent on cbp and protect against proteotoxicity. PLoS One. 2011;6(11):e27762.

Luders E, Clark K, Narr KL, Toga AW. Enhanced brain connectivity in long-term meditation practitioners. Neuroimage. 2011 Aug 15;57(4):1308-16.

Luders E, Toga AW, Lepore N, Gaser C. The underlying anatomical correlates of long-term meditation: larger hippocampal and frontal volumes of gray matter. Neuroimage. 2009 Apr 15;45(3):672-8.

Luke J. Fluoride deposition in the aged human pineal gland. Caries Res. 2001 Mar-Apr;35(2):125-8.

Lyte, M. Probiotics function mechanistically as delivery vehicles for neuroactive compounds: Microbial endocrinology in the design and use of probiotics. Bioessays. doi: 10.1002/bies.201100024

M Nakagawara. Beta-phenylethylamine and noradrenergic function in depression. Prog Neuropsychopharmacol Biol Psychiatry 16(1):45-53 (1992).

Marshall L, Born J. The contribution of sleep to hippocampus-dependent memory consolidation. Trends In Cognitive Sciences. 2007 Oct;11(10):442-50.

Mason, R. 200mg of Zen: Alternative and Complementary Therapies. Larchmont, NY: Mary Ann Liebert, Inc., 2001.

MØLLER Niels, OTTO Jens, JØRGENSEN Lunde. Effects of Growth Hormone on Glucose, Lipid, and Protein Metabolism in Human Subjects. Endocrine review. 2009 Apr;30(2):152-77. doi: 10.1210/er.2008-0027. Epub 2009 Feb 24.

Mu X, He GR, Yuan X, Li XX, Du GH. Baicalein protects the brain against neuron impairments induced by MPTP in C57BL/6 mice. Pharmacology, Biochemistry and Behavior. 2011 Apr;98(2):286-91.

Myerson, A., and Neustadt, R., 'Influence of Ultraviolet Irradiation upon Excretion of Sex Hormones In The Male', Endocrinology: 25; 7, 1939.

National Sleep Foundation: "How Much Sleep Do You Really Need?"

Native American Ethnobotany Database, University of Michigan Dearborne. Features a searchable database of medicinal uses of plant substances (including blueberries) in North America.

Nicola Reavley; The New Encyclopedia of Vitamins, Minerals, Supplements, and Herbs;1999

Owen RW, Haubner R, Würtele G, Hull E, Spiegelhalder B, Bartsch H. Olives and olive oil in cancer prevention. European Journal of Cancer Prevention. 2004 Aug;13(4):319-26.

P. Shekelle et al; AHRQ.gov; Effect of Supplemental Antioxidants Vitamin C, Vitamin E, and Coenzyme Q10 for the Prevention and Treatment of Cardiovascular Disease; 2003

Page KA, Williamson A, Yu N, McNay EC, Dzuira J, McCrimmon RJ, Sherwin RS. Medium-chain fatty acids improve cognitive function in intensively treated type 1 diabetic patients and support in vitro synaptic transmission during acute hypoglycemia. Diabetes. 2009 May;58(5):1237-44. doi: 10.2337/db08-1557. Epub 2009 Feb 17.

Papandreou MA, Dimakopoulou A, Linardaki ZI, Cordopatis P, Klimis-Zacas D, Margarity M, -Lamari FN. Effect of a polyphenol-rich wild blueberry extract on cognitive performance of mice, brain antioxidant markers and acetylcholinesterase activity. Behavioural Brain Research. 2009 Mar 17;198(2):352-8.

Penzel T, Möller M, Becker HF, Knaack L, Peter JH. Effect of sleep position and sleep stage on the collapsibility of the upper airways in patients with sleep apnea. Sleep. 2001 Feb 1;24(1):90-5.

Pérez RA, Iglesias MT, Pueyo E, Gonzalez M, de Lorenzo C. Amino acid composition and antioxidant capacity of Spanish honeys. J Agric Food Chem. 2007 Jan 24;55(2):360-5.

Phyllis A. Balch; "Prescription for Herbal Healing";CNC; 2002

Pogge E. Vitamin D and Alzheimer's disease: is there a link? The Consultant Pharmacist: The Journal of the American Society of Consultant Pharmacists. 2010 Jul;25(7):440-50.

Prediger, R., et al. "Effects of acute administration of the hydroalcoholic extract of mate tea leaves (Ilex para-guariensis) in animal models of learning and memory." J Ethnopharmacol. 2008 Dec 8;120(3):465-73.

Presley TD, Morgan AR, Bechtold E, Clodfelter W, Dove RW, Jennings JM, Kraft RA, King SB, Laurienti PJ, Rejeski WJ, Burdette JH, Kim-Shapiro DB,Miller GD. Acute effect of a high nitrate diet on brain perfusion in older adults. Nitric Oxide: Biology and Chemistry 2011 Jan 1;24(1):34-42.

Proceedings of The National Academy of Sciences of The United States of America. 2011 Feb 15;108(7):3017-22.

Przybelski RJ, Binkley NC. Is vitamin D important for preserving cognition? A positive correlation of serum

25-hydroxyvitamin D concentration with cognitive function. Arch Biochem Biophys. 2007 Apr 15;460(2):202-5.

R.L. Veech et. al; IUBMB Life; Ketone Bodies, Potential Therapeutic Uses; April 2001.

RajaSankar S, Manivasagam T, Sankar V, Prakash S, Muthusamy R, Krishnamurti A, Surendran S. Withania somnifera root extract improves catecholamines and physiological abnormalities seen in aParkinson's disease model mouse. Journal of Ethnopharmacol. 2009 Sep 25;125(3):369-73.

Ramanujan, K. "Satellite Sees Ocean Plants Increase, Coasts Greening". NASA. 2 March 2005. Retrieved 12 January 2009.

Rao, AV, et al;. A randomized, double-blind, placebo-controlled pilot study of a probiotic in emotional symptoms of chronic fatigue syndrome. GUT PATHOGENS. Vol 1, Num 1, 6. 19 Mar 2009. DOI: 10.1186/1757-4749-1-6

Rein G "Bio-information and non-local interactions between biological systems." Proc. Society for Scientific Exploration, Boulder, CO. June, 2011

Rein G. "The in vitro effect of bioenergy on the conformational states of human DNA in aqueous solutions" J. Acupuncture & Electrotherapeutics Res. 20: 173-180, 1995

Rein G. "Utilization of a New In-Vitro Bioassay to Quantify the Effects of Conscious Intention of Healing Practitioners"

The Science of Whole Person Healing, Vol.2, R.Roy (ed). Iuniverse Inc, Lincoln, NE, p222-236, 2003

Renata Viana Abreu, Eliane Moretto Silva-Oliveira, Márcio Flávio Dutra Moraes, Grace Schenatto Pereira, Tasso Moraes-Santos. Chronic coffee and caffeine ingestion effects on the cognitive function and antioxidant system of rat brains .Pharmacology Biochemistry and Behavior. Volume 99, Issue 4, October 2011, Pages 659–664.

Robert Mastone. "The Neuroscience of the Gut". Scientific American, April 19, 2011.

Robin McKie Warning: nicotine seriously improves health

Roodenrys S, Booth D, Bulzomi S, Phipps A, Micallef C, Smoker J. Chronic effects of Brahmi (Bacopa monnieri) on human memory. Neuropsychopharmacology. 2002 Aug;27(2):279-81.

Roseman, L. et al; Front Hum Neurosci. 2014; 8: 204. Published online May 27, 2014. doi: 10.3389/fnhum.2014.00204

Roseman, L. The effects of psilocybin and MDMA on between-network resting state functional connectivity in healthy volunteers;

Ross Fiziol Zh Im I M Sechenova. Possible mechanisms of learning, memory and attention impairment in consequence of sleep deprivation. 2012 Oct;98(10):1200-12.

S. Mahadevan, Y. Park; 2008"Journal of Food Science";

Multifaceted Therapeutic Benefits of Ginkgo biloba L.: Chemistry, Efficacy, Safety, and Uses; 2008

Salazar MJ, El Hafidi M, Pastelin G, Ramírez-Ortega MC, Sánchez-Mendoza MA. Effect of an avocado oil-rich diet over an angiotensin II-induced blood pressure response. Journal of Ethnopharmacol. 2005 Apr 26;98(3):335-8.

Schaffer, Sebastian, et al; Hydroxytyrosol-rich olive mill wastewater extract protects brain cells in vitro and ex vivo. Journal of Agricultural and Food Chemistry (impact factor: 2.82). 06/2007; 55(13):5043-9. DOI:10.1021/jf0703710

Sedriep S, Xia X, Marotta F, Zhou L, Yadav H, Yang H, Soresi V, Catanzaro R, Zhong K, Polimeni A, Chui DH. Beneficial nutraceutical modulation of cerebral erythropoietin expression and oxidative stress: an experimental study. J Biol Regul Homeost Agents. 2011 Apr-Jun;25(2):187-94.

Shergill, Amandeep (1998). "Ginseng and Memory". Nutrition Bytes 4 (2). Retrieved 4-3-2013.

Shevchuk NA. Adapted cold shower as a potential treatment for depression. Med Hypotheses. 2008;70(5):995-1001.

Shevtsov VA, Zholus BI, Shervarly VI, et al. (Mar 2003). "A randomized trial of two different doses of Rhodiola rosea extract versus placebo and control of capacity for mental work". Phytomedicine 10 (2–3): 95–105.

Shytle DR, Tan J, Ehrhart J, Smith AJ, Sanberg CD, Sanberg PR, Anderson J, Bickford PC. Effects of blue-green algae extracts on the proliferation of human adult stem cells in vitro: a preliminary study. Med Sci Monit. 2010 Jan;16(1):BR1-5.

Simon, H.; University of Maryland Medical Center; Vitamins Dietary Health Benefits; February 2009

Simonetti, G. (1990). Schuler, S.. ed. Simon & Schuster's Guide to Herbs and Spices. Simon & Schuster, Inc. ISBN 0-671-73489-X.

Snitz BE, et al; Ginkgo Evaluation of Memory (GEM) Study Investigators. Ginkgo biloba for preventing cognitive decline in older adults: a randomized trial. JAMA. 2009 Dec 23;302(24):2663-70.

Sokal K, Sokal P. Earthing the human organism influences bioelectrical processes. J Altern Complement Med. 2012 Mar;18(3):229-34. doi: 10.1089/acm.2010.0683.

Sokal K, Sokal P. Earthing the human organism influences bioelectrical processes. J Altern Complement Med. 2012 Mar;18(3):229-34. doi: 10.1089/acm.2010.0683.

Sokal P, Sokal K. The neuromodulative role of earthing. Med Hypotheses. 2011 Nov;77(5):824-6. doi: 10.1016/j.mehy.2011.07.046.

Sokal P, Sokal K. The neuromodulative role of earthing. Med Hypotheses. 2011 Nov;77(5):824-6. doi: 10.1016/j.mehy.2011.07.046.

Sorensen, H., and Sonne, J., A double-masked study of the effects of ginseng on cognitive functions, Current therapeutic research, clinical and experimental. 1996, 57:959–68.

Sreeramulu, Guttapadu; Zhu, Yang; Knol, Wieger (2000). "Kombucha Fermentation and Its Antimicrobial Activity". Journal of Agricultural and Food Chemistry 48(6): 2589–94.

Steiner, Rudolf; Lectures to Workers, Dornach, 18th July 1923.

Sudhanshu Saxena, Anjali Sahay,1 and Pankaj Goel. Effect of fluoride exposure on the intelligence of school children in Madhya Pradesh, India. J Neurosci Rural Pract. 2012 May-Aug; 3(2): 144–149.

Sumayayo, Marco. "What are the medicinal uses of San Pedro Cactus?" 30 July 2014. 2003-2014

Tees RC, Mohammadi E. The effects of neonatal choline dietary supplementation on adult spatial and configural learning and memory in rats. Developmental Psychobiology. 1999 Nov;35(3):226-40. The Observer. Sunday 18 July 2004. http://observer.theguardian.com/uk_news/story/0,6903,1263845,00.html

Tenney, Louise; Today's Herbal Health: The Essential Reference Guide; 2007

Tine Tholstrup, Christian Ehnholm, Matti Jauhiainen, et al.; "The American Journal of Clinical Nutrition"; Effects of Medium-Chain Fatty Acids and Oleic Acid on Blood Lipids, Lipoproteins, Glucose, Insulin, and Lipid Transfer Protein Activities; April 2004.

Tohda C, Kuboyama T, Komatsu K. Search for natural

products related to regeneration of the neuronal network. Neurosignals. 2005;14(1-2):34-45.

Tomkins, P. Bird, C. "The Secret life of Plants" (1973)

Tze-Pin Ng 1 , Peak-Chiang Chiam 2 , Theresa Lee 2 , Hong-Choon Chua 2 , Leslie Lim 3 and Ee-Heok Kua 1 Curry Consumption and Cognitive Function in the Elderly. Am. J. Epidemiol. (1 November 2006) 164 (9): 898-906.

Van Praag H, Christie BR, Sejnowski TJ, Gage FH. Running enhances neurogenesis, learning, and long-term potentiation in mice. Proceedings of The National Academy of Sciences of The United States of America. 1999 Nov 9;96(23):13427-31.

Vinod Gujral, Ph.D; Enviro-Health Research Laboratories; Marine Phytoplankton Certificate of Analysis.

Vinoo Alluri, Petri Toiviainen, Iiro P. Jääskeläinen, Enrico Glerean, Mikko Sams, Elvira Brattico. Large-scale brain networks emerge from dynamic processing of musical timbre, key and rhythm. NeuroImage, 2011; DOI:10.1016/j.neuroimage.2011.11.019

Volume 23, Issue 3, pages 255–e119, March 2011.

Webb AJ, Patel N, Loukogeorgakis S, Okorie M, Aboud Z, Misra S, Rashid R, Miall P, Deanfield J, Benjamin N, MacAllister R, Hobbs AJ, Ahluwalia A. "Acute blood pressure lowering, vasoprotective, and antiplatelet properties of dietary nitrate via bioconversion to nitrite." Hypertension. 2008 Mar;51(3):784-90.

Williams, Penry (1964). Life in Tudor England. Batsford. p. 88.

Wood, R."The New Whole Foods Encyclopedia"; 1999

Yang H, Jiang Y. [Research progress of bioactive constituents, absorption, metabolism, and neuroprotective effects from blueberry]. Wei Sheng Yan Jiu. 2010 Jul;39(4):525-8.

Yaryura-Tobias, J. A., Heller, B., Spatz, H., and Fischer, et al. : Phenylalanine for Endogenous Depression. J. Ortho. Psychiat. 3(21:80-81, 1974.

Yoon SY, Dela Peña I, Kim SM, Woo TS, Shin CY, Son KH, Park H, Lee YS, Ryu JH, Jin M, Kim KM, Cheong JH. Oroxylin A improves attention deficit hyperactivity disorder-like behaviors in the spontaneously hypertensive rat and inhibits reuptake of dopamine in vitro. Archives of Pharmacal Research. 2013 Jan;36(1):134-40.

Yousef GG, Grace MH, Cheng DM, Belolipov IV, Raskin I, Lila MA (Nov 2006). "Comparative phytochemical characterization of three Rhodiola species". Phytochemistry 67 (21): 2380–91.doi:10.1016/j.phytochem.2006.07.026.PMID 16956631.

Yu MS, Leung SK, Lai SW, Che CM, Zee SY, So KF, Yuen WH, Chang RC. Neuroprotective effects of anti-aging oriental medicine Lycium barbarum against beta-amyloid peptide neurotoxicity. Exp Gerontol. 2005 Aug-Sep;40(8-9):716-27.

Zamani Z, Reisi P, Alaei H, Pilehvarian AA. Effect of Royal Jelly on spatial learning and memory in rat model of streptozotocin-induced sporadic Alzheimer's disease. Advanced Biomedical Research. 2012;1:26. doi: 10.4103/2277-9175.98150. Epub 2012 Jul 6.

Zhou QB, Jia Q, Zhang Y, Li LY, Chi ZF, Liu P. "Effects of baicalin on protease-activated receptor-1 expression and brain injury in a rat model of intracerebral hemorrhage". The Chinese Journal of Physiology. 2012 Jun 30;55(3):202-9.

Zielińska-Przyjemska M, Olejnik A, Dobrowolska-Zachwieja A, Grajek W. "In vitro effects of beetroot juice and chips on oxidative metabolism and apoptosis in neutrophils from obese individuals." Phytotherapy Research 2009 Jan;23(1):49-55.

Made in the USA
Middletown, DE
15 January 2015